Just Fuck Me!

WHAT WOMEN WANT MEN TO KNOW ABOUT TAKING CONTROL IN THE BEDROOM

A GUIDE FOR COUPLES

Just Fuck Me!

What Women Want Men to Know About Taking Control in the Bedroom

A Guide for Couples

By Eve Kingsley

Published by

Secret Life Publishing

www.SecretLifePublishing.com

Contact info:

KRE Book Group
PO Box 121135
Nashville, TN 37212

Table of Contents

Part Three:
Tips and Suggestions For Couples (con't)

NOTE FROM THE AUTHOR

Several years ago, a friend of mine emailed me the day after his girlfriend broke up with him. He wanted a female perspective, to help him understand her reasons for ending their relationship, seemingly, out of the blue.

The thing that really threw him for a loop was her complaint that he didn't understand her sexual needs. She told him there were times, a lot of times, when she wanted to be "bent over and fucked hard" (her exact words), without the tenderness, extended foreplay, or romance that he thought she preferred.

"I didn't want her to feel disrespected," he wrote.

Our email exchange went on for a week—him asking for clarity and me giving advice and doing my best to explain that, yes, sometimes women want men to get aggressive in the bedroom.

I started thinking more about the topic...and asked both female and male friends for their opinions on it. To my surprise, quite often, the women I talked with were frustrated that men didn't sense those times when they wanted to bypass "making love" and get straight to "fucking."

And many of the men I spoke with were both perplexed and frustrated, because they could never seem to accurately read what their partners wanted and when they wanted it.

But here's what really shocked me...

Men and women weren't talking to each other about this!

I told a writer friend about what I'd come to realize.

He said, "You'd think talking openly would be the obvious solution, but sometimes people just don't know how. Someone should write a book to teach them."

That's how the idea for the original version of this book came to be.

What you're about to read is the newly revised (and expanded) edition, with the collected wisdom of my own experiences from years as a relationship coach, as well as those of you who read the original book and offered your perspective on how it could be improved.

Some people, maybe you, have picked up this book as a novelty item. The subject is anything but "novelty" though. When it comes to the topic of improving male-female communication, I'm *very* serious. I've worked with thousands of couples over the years and seen how devastating unspoken sexual desires can be-- not just to a relationship, but to each individual's own well-being.

Still, this book is not for everybody and it may not be for you. In order for you to receive total benefit from what I'm talking about, you (as well as your partner) will have to approach things with an open mind and you'll have to be willing to change up the parts of your relationship that aren't working.

You'll have to be vulnerable.

Is that scary? Hell yes, it's scary.

Being able to take a risk and ask for what you want might be one of the hardest things you'll ever do, but it can also lead you to the most rewarding and sexually satisfying experiences of your life.

To me, that's worth the risk!

Congratulations on taking your relationship to the next level!

Eve

INTRODUCTION

There is a secret bit of fun that most women are too shy to admit, most men are too scared to try, and most of the couples who practice it don't ever talk about outside the bedroom. It's not that kinky or crazy, and it's something that recent polls have shown drive women wild.

What is it? It's that more and more women long to be sexually dominated. They want alpha males, assertive and strong, taking charge of their nocturnal activities.

It doesn't sound like such an outlandish thing to talk about, I know. But, more often than not, women are afraid to ask their men to be a bit rougher in the bedroom – and men get remarkably timid when they feel they're crossing the line when it comes to dominating their sexual partners.

This is understandable. In the last few decades, there has been a combination of the feminist revolution and the birth of political correctness. And, sadly, there are still too many women out there who have been raped, sexually abused or assaulted by men – and more often than not, by men they know and with whom they have intimate relationships.

So, it's entirely within the realm of reason that a woman who feels any sort of kinship with feminism and the female power dynamic would be reluctant to ask her man to be more ... well ... "manly" in the bedroom. And, a man who respects his woman is not going to jump at the chance to treat her like she's any less than he.

It can be scary to entertain the thought of voluntarily being roughed up during sex – just as it can be intimidating to be the one doing the roughing up. Surely, both have concerns:

- Does she really want this?
- How assertive can I be?

- Am I pushing it too far?
- Am I being assertive enough?
- Will he be able to stop?
- Is this what he wants?
- Is this what she wants?
- How will he treat me outside the bedroom?
- Will this change our relationship?
- How do I bring this up with him in the first place?
- What happens when I want it to stop?
- Isn't it too crazy to want to do this?

But, it doesn't have to be this way. Male domination in the bedroom is a perfectly normal fantasy shared by millions of couples in healthy, long-term, loving relationships. It's so common that it's not even on the same scale as role-playing, or BDSM techniques, or anything that would require a great deal of effort.

Think of it this way: on the scale of kink, having your man be rough and manly with you doesn't even tip the balance. To put your fantasy into perspective, consider this:

- There are successful executives who like to wear diapers and be spanked.
- There are couples that only have sexual relations when dressed up as large stuffed animals.
- There are couples that are aroused only when others are watching them.
- Some men like to be forced to wear women's clothing, or to lick their wife's shoes.
- Some women like to pee on their partner during sex.

So, you see, couples that like a little rough sex every once in a while really aren't pushing the envelope on the kink factor. It's a perfectly normal impulse for women, and it's absolutely fine for men to want to make this fantasy come true.

By the time you finish reading this book, both of you will feel comfortable enough to talk about your bedroom desires, and to start to act out some male-dominant scenarios during your next trip to the bedroom.

*** *** ***

The first part of this book is for the men. Any guy worth his salt is going to be apprehensive about roughing up his partner during loving, consensual sex. Hopefully, this book will answer any questions you have about this type of fantasy, and how you can be successful at indulging your ladylove – starting tonight!

Ladies, the second part of this book is dedicated to you. Together, we'll help you figure out exactly what it is you want your man to do in the bedroom, how to talk to him about it, and how to show him, too. We'll discuss the boundaries you should set up, and we'll also talk about what this does and doesn't mean for you outside the bedroom.

The last section of this book should be read and talked about by the both of you, as it provides tips and suggestions for couples to get into the spirit of the woman's desires. We'll cover dirty talk, rough intercourse, how to take it up a notch and what toys or games can be brought into the mix for a little fun – or even to just get started.

I'm thrilled to be able to share my knowledge about this exciting, intimate sex play that makes so many couples around the world feel closer. Now, if you're both ready, this is the time to hand the book over to the "manly man" of the house. It's time to get started!

PART ONE:

FOR **MEN**

SHE LIKES IT ROUGH? REALLY?

Oh, guys, guys, guys. I can only imagine how confusing this must be for you. I don't blame you – finding out your woman wants you to be a "caveman" and rough it up a bit goes against pretty much everything you know.

First of all, it goes against how you were probably raised. Even if your dad was a lumberjack when you were a kid, just think for a moment about all the advice you've gotten in your life, from when you were just a little tyke:

- Respect your mother.
- Be gentle with your sister.
- You can't hit girls.
- Girls hate bullies.
- You need to be a nice guy if you want to find a decent girl.
- Call her Ma'am, or Miss.
- Open doors for ladies.

The list goes on and on. Then, when you grew up – and so did the women around you – there came terrifying concepts like date rape and sexual harassment. I'm sure at your college or at your job you've attended a mandatory training session about what is and is not acceptable with women in more formal settings:

- No lewd jokes.
- No touching.
- No complimenting.
- No dating in the workplace.

And that's on top of the fight women have had for equality, of which I'm sure you're well aware. Unlike the generations before you, you've probably had at least one female boss, or at least know women who make more money than you or are in higher positions in your field of work. So, it's been drummed into your head that:

- Women are just as good at tough jobs as men.
- Women deserve equal pay.
- Women can assume positions of authority.
- Women must be treated with the same respect as men.

And dating is another whole kettle of fish, isn't it? Seriously, how much advice have you received over the years about dating and relationships? How many magazine polls have you read? How many times have you pulled one of your friends aside and asked them for help with a girl?

And, what have you learned?

- Treat your woman well.
- Respect your woman.
- Do everything you can to make your woman feel appreciated.
- Make sure your woman knows she's important to you.

- NO means NO.
- And, of course, when it comes to sex, there is an entire universe of things to remember in order to please your partner:
- Be gentle.
- Follow your woman's lead.
- Your priority should be pleasing her.
- Women like to be romanced a bit.
- It's not just "Wham, bam! Thank you, Ma'am.

Taking this lifetime of advice into account, you've become a man who understands women better, treats women with more respect, and is more in tune with his partner than at any other time in modern relationship history. You finally feel like you've gotten it right – and you and the ladylove of your life have never been happier.

But then you find out that your woman wants you to be an alpha male. What the hell are you supposed to do with this ticking bomb of information she's laid at your feet? What does she even mean?

Take a breath. Relax. That's why you're reading this book. We'll figure it all out together, and get you on the road to having the best sex of your life with the woman you adore.

*** *** ***

Obviously, having great sex and exploring your sexual side is an important part of your relationship. But this book has absolutely nothing to do with how you relate to each other on a day-to-day basis. This is not a relationship advice book. This is a guide to pleasing your woman in bed.

So, let's talk about sex!

WHY BEING AN ALPHA MALE IS SUCH A TURN-ON FOR WOMEN

The first question you probably have is, *Why do women want men to be sexually assertive?*

The answer to this can be incredibly complex. And while every woman brings her own unique perspective to the table when it comes to sexual relationships, there are a few common reasons why women like men who are more assertive in the bedroom.

Surprisingly, one broad-stroke reason is feminism.

WHAT?! I know. *How could something that inspires a woman to be strong and in control also be behind her desire for an alpha male in the bedroom?*

It might be hard for you to truly grasp what a day in the life of a woman is like. But, let me tell you, it ain't easy. For so many women, each day is filled with worries, struggles, slights, plans, maneuvering – you name it, and they have to find a way to handle it during the course of their day. In addition, these things double in intensity when she's dealing with men in any capacity.

If you are still not convinced that women have it hard, consider these examples:

- The woman who thinks life is just dandy, and never has a problem getting what she wants – especially from men. Little does she know, the very essence of her personality is derived from how she perceives the world perceives her, and she's learned how to work it.

- The woman who has been a bridesmaid 14 times in the last two years, and has had to find lighthearted answers every time she is asked when it'll be her turn to walk down the aisle.

- The woman who gives a detailed opinion about Madonna's marriages, divorces, fitness regimen and mothering skills – because she feels she has to have an opinion, otherwise people might think she feels touchy about aging.
- The woman who really loves her career, and doesn't feel the need to be in a relationship – or the woman who loves being a stay-at-home mom.
- The girl who wants to wait until she's married to have sex – or the girl who really, really doesn't want to wait even one more second.

Do you see the complex issues involved with being a woman? Yes, that includes your woman as well. So sometimes, at the end of the day, a woman just wants to be ravished by her man. She wants to shed that hard defensive shell she's had to lug around all day and lose control in the arms of the man she loves.

Here's an analogy for a woman's desire: It's like how Ed Norton's character feels in the movie *Fight Club*. He's just so beaten down by everything about his life, as well as the expectations he is supposed to live up to, that he finds a kind of release and purity in participating in the fight club. It's a strange correlation, I know, but it's that core emotion that is similar to what your woman feels.

Another reason she wants you to be more assertive: it's a normal impulse. Men don't come anywhere near realizing this impulse in themselves (i.e. the impulse of wanting to be dominated) because they tend to be stopped by the fear of seeming weak – something that has been drilled into them since they were little.

But it's a perfectly natural thing. Just as sometimes she likes to get on top, ride you like a bronco and call all the shots, so too does she sometimes want you to show her who's the boss of your bedroom.

Honestly, testing your sexual control is a healthy part of any solid sexual relationship. You probably have already done this on a more subtle level; now, your woman wants you to kick it up a notch.

One more general reason has to do with a combination of feminist reaction and assertiveness. It's about your woman's sexuality, and how she perceives the power of her own beauty and confidence.

Whenever your woman buys a new piece of clothing, a new kind of makeup or gets her hair cut or colored, she is rethinking her appearance and testing the boundaries of what she considers to be beautiful. She's seeing how far she can go to show her beauty to others, while still maintaining her dignity, in a manner of speaking, and a solid sense of self.

It is this notion – the conscious objectification of herself – that can make almost any woman feel a rush of animal-like arousal. It's her taking control of her sexuality by using it as a tool. By appearing more feminine and beautiful, she is also feeling more powerful.

I know it sounds weird. And I realize that it might be a confusing idea to men, who walk into a store, pull a pair of pants or a shirt in their size off the rack, pay for it and leave the store without a second thought. But really, it's that single moment of primal sexuality that can lead a woman to want to experiment with it in the bedroom too.

WHAT IS AN ALPHA MALE?

So, what is an "alpha male"? Simply put, an alpha male is a man's man. He is someone who exudes masculinity. Someone who looks like they'd be a challenge in a fight. A man who is all man, inside and out.

Does that mean an alpha male is one of those ex-frat-boy douche bags who still thinks he's on the high school football team?

Well, to be honest, sometimes it is. There is a definite bulldog, I'm-the-man-here quality to that type of guy. And there are girls who are attracted to that type of guy.

But for the vast majority of women, there is something decidedly unattractive about this kind of alpha male. There is a certain vibe that comes off a guy like that; maybe he doesn't know when to set aside his alpha, or maybe he uses his alpha for the wrong reasons. But whatever it is, a douche bag alpha male is not particularly attractive to most women.

The ability to bench-press more than his body weight does not make a guy an alpha male. Again, there are women who are attracted to men whose muscles can barely be contained by their shirt. But more often than not, their vanity gets in the way of them appearing attractive to women.

An alpha male doesn't have to be the hottest guy in the room, either. Millions of women around the world fell in love with Leonardo DiCaprio as Jack in *Titanic*; and even today, Johnny Depp continues to capture female hearts aplenty. Even men can see their attractive qualities. But alpha men, they're not. Usually, famous alpha men are the ones whom men admire, too. So as not to betray my own preferences when it comes to movie stars, think back to men like Clint Eastwood, John Wayne and even Gene Hackman. None of them are necessarily sex symbols, but no one can doubt that they were MEN.

Or, let's talk about TV characters. It's Don Draper, not Peter Campbell, from *Mad Men*. Jack, not Charlie, from *Lost*. Josh Lyman, not Sam Seaborne, from *The West Wing*.

An alpha male has an indefinable quality that makes women of every stripe want to literally lie down for him. It's a take-control vibe. It's an "I can handle it" vibe. It's an "I'm the man, and you are the woman" vibe that, despite its sexist overtones, can still convey a sincere sense of respect for the fairer sex. It's a man who will break up a fight without throwing a punch, or whom you believe 100 percent when he says that everything is going to be all right.

Unless your relationship is severely dysfunctional, your woman is with you because at some point, and on some level neither of you might even be aware of, you exuded this alpha male quality. However, no matter how consistently you are an alpha male in your day-to-day relationship, there remains the fact that sometimes, it simply doesn't translate over to the bedroom as effectively as your woman would like.

This can be for a variety of reasons, none of which are deal breakers, and absolutely none of which are anyone's fault. Let's go over some of these reasons now, and see if maybe you can recognize yourself in these examples.

Sometimes, if a man is inexperienced sexually, there might me a few ways in which he is not responding to his partner's desires. He might be timid in the bedroom out of a fear of doing something wrong. It can be tough to know exactly how to please a woman in bed if you don't have a lot of experience in this area.

Also, inexperience sometimes correlates with an inability to read the signs a woman might be giving her partner that she wants to do certain things, or wants her partner to behave a certain way. It can be intimidating for a woman to come right out and say, "Slam me up against that wall and have sex with me while standing up!" But she might utter an excited cry, or say "Yes," and her partner might not be experienced enough to equate that directly to what he is or isn't doing and act on it further.

For more experienced men, there might be some confusion in their bedroom tactics that can lead to his partner's dissatisfaction. They say women are like snowflakes – no two are alike – and that couldn't be truer than in the bedroom.

So, if a man tried something with one woman, and she loved it, he might try it with another who hates it and runs out of the bedroom. That might be an extreme example of a woman's reaction – but it's not too far off the mark in terms of the visceral reaction women have while they're making love and are brought abruptly into or out of "the zone."

The problem this type of man has is that he's using a general tactic for all women, instead of paying attention to the woman who is with him right here, right now. He's not reading the signs during their lovemaking, and he's not taking into account the kind of woman she is outside of the bedroom as well.

This can lead to both partners being on different wavelengths while having sex – and that's not good for anybody! Men have to know how to read their women in bed.

Just because she says she wants you to be more assertive, that doesn't necessarily mean all the time. So if she's in a romantic mood, it's probably not the best moment to pull her hair. Likewise, if she's breathing hard and scratching your back and being rough with you, and you respond by taking her face in her hands and kissing her gently while you're inside of her, you're missing the mark.

This can be incredibly frustrating for a woman, especially if she is not used to having to explain herself in the bedroom. And, in the case of consensual sexual aggression, it might be hard for her to talk about it outright.

THE ART OF BEING ASSERTIVE

I know you love your lady, and you want her to be open and honest with you. But in the case of asking you to be assertive, there can be all kinds of conflicting feelings going on inside of her, and she's not quite sure how to broach the subject in a way that wouldn't completely freak you out.

Put it this way: Think about getting a blowjob. (Hey! Stay with me here.) A blowjob just plain feels good, right? It's not necessarily about love, admiration, mutual respect or any of the other things that makes your life with her so amazing. It's a blowjob.

But there can also be another element to a blowjob – the one in which you recognize that the woman you love is servicing you. There's little to no sexual arousal for a woman giving a blowjob – and if a woman tells you differently, she's doing so to make you feel good because she knows you might feel a bit guilty about the pleasure you derive from such an act.

So let's say you wanted to ask your wife or girlfriend to give you more blowjobs. Do you just come right out and say it? What if it makes her feel inferior, or like a bad sexual partner? What if she tells you to go to hell? What if she becomes convinced that you only like them because it puts you in a superior position?

You can see how you might feel conflicted about that. Well, it's the same with women – only reversed. In effect, she is asking you to treat her like a sexual object, to maybe talk to her like she's a whore, or maybe to get physically aggressive with her. You can only imagine the confusion she's feeling about how to approach you with such a request.

She's anxious. She doesn't want to talk about it for hours, because that will kill the mood once you eventually do try it in the bedroom. She wants to make sure you understand that it's ONLY in the bedroom; then she feels bad, because of course you would realize that; then she feels anxious again, because what if you don't? What if you reject her idea, and think she's some kind of freak?

There is a lot going on in that pretty little head of hers, and she's not telling you any of it right now.

For a certain kind of woman, there's also the issue of speaking up when it comes to sexual requests in general. She might not even know exactly what it is she wants, but she knows she's been frustrated in bed lately. However, she's simply not able to put words to the feeling she has – nor is she able to follow her own thought processes enough to get to a point that might seem extreme or taboo for her.

But every woman, even the most sexually inexperienced, finds ways to let you know what she does and doesn't like about your bedroom techniques. It's up to you to be able to read the clues, and act on them.

The key is to be aware when there is a change in her breathing, her rhythm, the way she speaks, her physical movements in relation to your body, and the general vibe she's giving off. Think about what you're doing at the moment you sense a different reaction in her, store it away for future use, and become that man she knows you can be.

- How did the sex initiate? Had you planned beforehand to have sex? Was it after a romantic evening out? Did she come in the door from work, take your hand and lead you into the bedroom? Did it seem to come out of nowhere for both of you?
- What kind of things is she doing to you? Is she leaving marks in your

back? Is she lazily playing with your hair? Is she biting your shoulder? Is she kissing you deeply, for a long time? Is she nuzzling gently in your neck?

- How is she reacting to what you're doing to her? Is she locking her eyes with yours and giving you hot looks? Does she seem lost in her own world? Does she pant and say, "Yes!" or kind of give you a kiss and send you on your way to an orgasm?

And speaking of orgasms, let's talk about them for a moment. I'm going to move past all the clichés about faking it, and just give you the truth – your woman has probably faked an orgasm with you.

Now, that's not necessarily a reflection on you. Because women don't need to have a physical reaction in order to have sex, it can be easier for them to simply allow sex to happen, without being particularly engaged in it – and this holds doubly true for women in relationships. We love you guys, and we know that when you're feeling particularly randy, it's better to have sex with you than to watch you behave like an injured puppy dog.

Or, it could be that she is really into the sex you're having, but her body is telling her otherwise. Trust me when I tell you how frustrating that can be. When this happens, it can be easier simply to fake an orgasm and be done with it than to make you go through a whole production to try to achieve something we know is not going to happen. It's also less awkward than telling you simply to stop, because we're aware of how that might be misconstrued when it's really not your fault at all.

The other reason why women fake orgasms is because they know there is just no way on earth you're going to get them to have one. Your timing is off, your technique is not doing it for them or you're simply not working in the sexual compatibility zone in that moment. This is not necessarily your fault. In fact, most times it's not your fault at all! But it does happen, and again, it's simply easier to fake it.

I'm going to give you some tips that can help you figure out if your woman is dissatisfied in the bedroom.

1. **Porn noises.** If your woman is naturally vocal in bed, I assure you those noises are involuntarily, even if she's aware she's making them. Therefore, I suggest you listen to them. If they're not sounding like their usual pitch, or tone or if she's sounding more like

a porn star than like a woman in the throes of passion, she's faking it.

2. **Pushing your buttons.** In any long-term relationship, each partner knows one little trick that immediately sets the other person into a tailspin of pleasure that crash lands in orgasm. If out of the blue she pulls out all the stops to get you to come, it's usually because she's ready for the sex to be over but she loves you enough not to push you off and get out of bed.
3. **"Silent" orgasms.** There you are, having sex with your ladylove, and all of a sudden you feel that she's kind of just lying there. Ask her, and she'll say she's had an orgasm, and is spent. In truth, she's done having sex, and is lying to you.
4. **LOUD orgasms.** If your partner sounds like Meg Ryan in the deli scene of *When Harry Met Sally*, she's faking it. You see, there is a place from where orgasm sounds come, and it's not a place one would call upon consciously. Note also, if loud orgasms make you orgasm, that's a win in her book. If she comes, and then you come, and she hops out of bed to check her email or walk the dog, she faked it.

HOW TO SATISFY HER (ALPHA MALE STYLE)

Now that I've got you all hyped up and extremely aware of the need to please your woman, let's go about succeeding at it. Let's get down to brass tacks.

I'm going to appeal to your problem-fixing nature and give you some serious, real-world tips on knowing your woman better, figuring out how to satisfy her and experimenting with your new-found sexual assertiveness. Fasten your seat belt!

If your partner has said absolutely nothing to you about it, but you want to find out if she wants you to be more sexually assertive, there are two ways to play it so that you'll have a pretty good idea. One of them is relatively easy; the other one, as far as I know, might be one of the most difficult things you've ever tried in bed.

The easier way, although it might be difficult for you at the start, is to plan out, all by yourself, a "spontaneous" moment of passion.

This can be pretty tricky. You want to catch her off guard and see how she reacts to your passionate ravishing, but you don't want to choose a time when she's going to glare at you and ask you if you have lost your mind.

In the interest of clarity, I'll go ahead and give you some straightforward pointers on the right and wrong times.

Right time: Immediately after you get home from a formal function. She's feeling devastatingly beautiful, you're looking fine, and you've been in a relatively uptight setting all night. Drop some hints about how much you want her throughout the evening. If she bites, start making out heavily as soon as you get your key in the door – or even sooner, maybe in the car on the way home. If she tells you to shut up or gives you the "knock it off" look when you're dropping your hints, let it go and try another time. She might be feeling a bit too uptight, particularly if it is her family you're with at the function.

Wrong time: When she's in grungy clothes and cleaning or organizing anything in the house. Stay away.

Wrong time: After your boys' night out. She's going to think you saw some hot chick and got all randy.

Toss-up: After her night out with the girls. If it was a bitching session, she's feeling the sister love and will not want to be manhandled by you. But, the bitching session might remind her why she loves you so much, and she'll want you to be the big man in her life and whisk her into the bedroom. Also, she might have been prowling around with her girls and is feeling gorgeous and sexy, and will want to be ravished by you. You're going to have to feel this one out on your own.

Right time: This one works if you're a bit shy. When you're in the house together, doing something together, you can start talking about how much you love it when you do whatever it is you're doing – but from a passionate perspective. This is a way to let a romantic notion become the impetus for a passionate, assertive move on your part. Talk about how much it turns you on that you're this great couple that's solid, and you love how much you can depend on that, and how nothing turns you on more than when you're doing things together in the house, because it makes you think about growing old with her ... you get the idea. Take her in your arms, be passionate, and be all man as you whisk her away to the bedroom. Sounds weird, I know, but it taps into the true alpha male vibe we love. (Something about you being the manly man provider who loves home and hearth.)

Wrong time: After you've had any kind of relationship discussion, argument or disagreement of any kind. She's going to see it as a power move, and not the kind that turns her on! Or, she'll see it as your way of apologizing, and she'll complain that sex doesn't solve everything.

Do you get the idea here? The right times are when you are on the same wavelength, are communicating well and are feeling that spark of true love for each other. The wrong times are when you're misreading her vibes, not aware of what she might be thinking, or while the air is still thick with disagreement.

By initiating a bit of spontaneous sexual activity – whether it's a hot make-out session, oral pleasure or full-on intercourse – you're able to show some sexual assertiveness to which she will definitely respond. What you need to watch out for is *how*.

If she rejects you outright, laugh it off and joke about how you'll get her later, or that she's all yours in bed tonight. Make an alpha male comment – now is not the time to apologize like you've done something seriously wrong.

If she lets you lead her, but she doesn't seem over-enthusiastic, she's "giving you" sex. It's something that women do sometimes; we know that men have different needs, and approach sex from a different point of view. Therefore, there are times we're phoning it in because we know you're simply responding to a sexual need.

I know that little bombshell may come as a surprise to some of you guys, but for the overwhelming majority of women, it rings very true. Don't dwell on it; but recognize the signs, because it will tell you if your partner is misreading your attempts at assertiveness.

Finally, if she franttically undresses and is grabbing at your clothes and has a monster of an orgasm – she's into it, and you should keep the spontaneous vibe going and add to it with some dominating moves (which we'll go over in a later section of this book).

When you are on the same wavelength, both of you will be much more open to trying new things – and not too upset if they don't turn out as titillating as either of you had hoped. We'll talk more about rejection below, but for now I want to get onto that second thing – the one I said might be the most difficult thing you've ever tried.

It requires me giving away one of "our" secrets!

You know that moment, oh, I don't know, about 30 seconds before you're about to have an orgasm? When your thrusts get that much deeper, that much harder, that much faster? When your mind falls off a cliff into oblivion?

Well, we love that part. And if your girl wants you to get rough, those 30 seconds are your window of opportunity to find out.

You see, we know you kind of lose it during that time. And if you want to be a bit rough – if you want to pull her hair, or smack her ass, or grab her breasts particularly hard, she's going to let you do it in that moment if she has an ounce of love for you in her heart.

They key is, though – and this is the hard part – is to see how she reacts. Does she let you do what you're doing because she knows what's coming, no pun intended? Or does she whole-heartedly join in, grabbing you and gritting her teeth and maybe biting you a bit? Does she have an instant orgasm right along with you? If it's the latter, you have a green light to talk to her about experimenting with assertiveness.

*** *** ***

When trying tactics like the ones above, or any other experimentation in the bedroom, there is bound to be some level of rejection, no matter how small. This is perfectly normal, and should not be taken as a reflection on you or your skills as a lover.

Even when you choose the right time and you're feeling the love, you still might be rejected outright. Hey, women are like snowflakes, remember?

But the fear of rejection can be a powerful motivator to do absolutely nothing – and that's the worst. Don't let your fear of rejection keep you from making what you feel is a bold, assertive move – from reaching over and kissing her, to being her dream man in the bedroom.

The most important thing here is that you only do what feels comfortable for you. Confidence in the bedroom is key – and if you're trying out a whole bunch of wacko stuff that makes you feel uncomfortable, weird or at all unlike yourself, she's going to sense that and close up like a clam. Literally.

The thing to keep in mind, in order to keep that confidence high, is that what happens in the bedroom is about your mutual pleasure. They don't call it "making love" just to be cheesy and embarrass you. For loving couples, sex of every stripe is the expression of the love you feel for each other. There's no need to hide from that. Sex is as natural as anything else on this earth, and your confidence in that fact will help you by leaps and bounds when you're getting it on.

Also, when your confidence is high, you're going to be more relaxed with your partner. When you're more relaxed, you're going to be more in tune with what she wants, and less worried about it – which is good, since worrying will get you exactly nowhere.

WHERE COMMUNICATION COMES INTO PLAY

Once you've tried out some of your more assertive moves during sex, it's a good idea to see how she feels about it, and most importantly, to ensure she's being honest with you. Communication is crucial when it comes to this kind of sexual experimentation. Even if your girl wants it bad, it can come with a lot of mental and emotional baggage. So to make it work in the bedroom, some things have to be addressed *outside* the bedroom.

But you don't want it to be like you're having an operational debriefing! Keep the excitement and the passion alive, even when you're talking about it. If she's really not into it, you'll know soon enough.

And if she's not really into it, talk about it as openly as you can, and be understanding. Even when it was her idea; even if it seemed like she enjoyed it at the time, she might be uncomfortable after she's thought about it a bit. Your job is to provide a safe, comfortable environment in which she can talk about how she feels.

And being supportive is important, too. She might not know how to express herself, so ask gentle questions that can kind of lead her through what she's thinking.

Communication while you're in bed is a tricky thing, but it can go far. There is something about combining communication with passion that can get the message across to each other in a way a "normal" conversation can't.

For example, say you've agreed to experiment with some assertive control. If you're both on the same wavelength, there can be a real give and take that can be actually quite exciting; a bit of, "You like that? You want it rougher, baby? You want me to call you a slut, is that what you want?" Can be replied to by a "Yes, yes, YES!" or an equally breathless and hot "No, give it to me slow now, Sugar. Nice and smooth," or "Tell me you love me, tell me I'm your baby."

I hope that example didn't make you nervous! Let's backtrack a moment and talk about what exactly sexual assertiveness is all about – and more importantly, what it isn't.

Right off the bat, I'll tell you that it has absolutely NOTHING to do with physical abuse. Not one thing. Nor is it about being an asshole. Instead, it is about taking control and calling the shots in the bedroom.

Now, within that framework, there is a lot of room for interpretation. It can mean anything from simply being the one who initiates sex, to telling your partner exactly what you want to do to her or what you want her to do to you, to spanking, biting and hair-pulling. It's all a matter of degrees, and it all depends on what you as a couple are comfortable doing. Not everyone has to swing from the chandeliers!

One more thing it isn't: BAD or WEIRD. Sex, and all sexual activity, is comprised of a powerful dynamic between you and your partner. To experiment with sexual assertiveness is a perfectly natural thing to do, as it shows you are observing that dynamic and wanting to explore your boundaries.

Likewise, as we have gone over previously, there are many, many reasons why your partner wants you to be more sexually assertive.

Once you come to terms with this dynamic, your next step is to overcome any shyness you have, or any fear you have of being assertive, and to go ahead and come out of that shell and show your lady you're all man!

OVERCOMING SHYNESS

So, let's talk about overcoming that shyness of yours.

It's perfectly OK to be shy when it comes to sex. There are many perfectly normal reasons why.

- You might not love the way your body's looking right now.
- You've been feeling unconnected with your wife or girlfriend.
- You're not sexually experienced.
- You had a bit of equipment malfunction recently, and you are afraid it'll happen again.
- Something embarrassing happened the last time you had sex.
- It's been a while since you two have gotten it on.
- You're distracted by work stress, relationship tension, or maybe you're not getting along with a friend.
- You really want to have sex, but you're not getting the "please jump me" vibe from your better half.

That's just a partial list. My point is that it's totally OK to be feeling shy about having any sex at all, let alone any kind of experimental sex. But let's see if we can come up with some ideas to get you back to taking care of business.

The key is not to think about the actual sex part. Work your way up to that by gaining your confidence in other ways.

- Start by being more physical with her during non-sexual times; a hand on the back when letting her go in front of you, a touch as you pass in the hallway or the kitchen, or taking her hand or linking arms when you're walking together.
- Kiss her! There are a million ways to kiss her. Don't be apologetic or shy about taking a moment to spin her around, take her in your arms and kiss her. It'll make you feel less shy, and it'll boost your alpha male status! Especially if you tell her it's for no reason except that she's your woman and she's beautiful.
- Waiting in line at the movies? Standing at the kitchen sink? Reading at the table? Use these times to bear hug her from behind and give a little nuzzle. Again, it will make you more com-

fortable being physical, and asserting yourself with her.

- To kick it up a notch and get you back in the game, go for some light making out when there's no chance of it leading to sex – in the car before going into a restaurant, in the hallway by the bathrooms at the bar, or just about anyplace else you can think of that wouldn't make either of you uncomfortable or embarrassed. It even works at home!

This last one also works as you get more confident for showing a little bit more assertiveness. If she starts to pull away a bit, pull her closer and keep going a little bit longer than she wants – you decide when it's time to stop.

As for getting down in the sack, lengthy foreplay is best to overcome shyness. Make out like it's your job! Make out until neither of you can stand it anymore. Even if she seems overly ready to take it to the next level, tell her you're not done with her yet, and really drive her wild.

When you're both super ready to have sex, shyness will be the last thing on your mind, I assure you. It will also boost your confidence to have a woman begging you to be inside her! And you will have found another way to start moving in on alpha male territory in the bedroom.

I'd like to say a word or two about talking to your partner about your shyness. Obviously, this might be difficult to do! And to be honest, while I advocate open communication, sometimes talking about shyness in the bedroom can make it become a much larger issue than it needs to be.

If you do feel the need to talk about it, I'd recommend doing it right after having sex. This might sound strange, I know, but it's a good time to open up about the feelings you're having. This can also start a discussion about how she can help you work it out, which is a wonderful time to bring up assertiveness. You can tell her what you want to have happen during your next roll in the hay, and you can get around to calling the shots in a way that completely has her on your side.

MAKING IT A HOT, PASSIONATE EXPERIENCE SHE WILL REMEMBER

Later on in this book, I'm going to talk to you about the specifics of alpha male bedroom behavior. But for now, I'd like to address how to communicate in the bedroom in a way that makes you both feel comfortable without blowing the whole vibe.

Real-time demonstrating and reinforcement are two ways to keep the mood while figuring out if what you're doing is working or not. Let's take a look at what that means.

Some people mistakenly think that male assertiveness in the bedroom is the equivalent of "Bitch, make me a sandwich." This couldn't be further from the truth. As I've said before, I want to stress that this has nothing to do with the fact that equality is the foundation of any strong relationship.

When you're experimenting with assertiveness in the bedroom, however, it's important to communicate with your partner. This lets her know what you're up to, and that you're not going overboard. It also allows her to have the confidence to speak up if she's uncomfortable.

A way to do this while keeping things hot and getting her involved is by demonstration. For example, say you want her to give you a blowjob in a particular way. Instead of explaining it, tell her you want a blowjob "like this" – and then go down on her to show her the rhythm or tongue trick you might want. This makes it a mutual pleasure-seeking activity while playing the assertive role.

Another example of staying in the moment while making subtle adjustments or directing what's going on is when she's uncomfortable with something you're doing. Say you're having "doggie-style" sex and you're pulling her hair, and she says "OUCH!" in a way that is not part of the sexy vibe. Don't panic – the mood isn't ruined! Stop pulling, but instead run your fingers through her hair. Then, gradually build back up to pulling, but not so tight. And no need to fumble or apologize; a simple, "OK, Baby" will suffice. Use your actions more than words or explanations, and you'll soon see you will have developed a language all your own.

A debriefing afterward doesn't have to be so clinical, either. Keep the talk brief and in the moment still. Instead of saying, "I hope I wasn't too rough" or apologizing for something she hasn't even brought up, keep a subtle air of alpha male where this is concerned.

"How about when I did this or that, was that too rough for you, Baby? You just say the word, and I'll be all over you. Damn, that was hot." Let her know that it's a mutual pleasure that is derived from this experimentation, while making it clear that even though you're in charge, it's all being done in a safe environment.

There can be a situation where, once you've gotten into acting out this scenario, you are, or she is, simply not into it. Or, the both of you might take one look at each other and say, "This is ridiculous."

This is OK, and perfectly normal. Not everything works for everyone. But, it's important to keep the lines of communication open so there is no misunderstanding about why this particular thing isn't working.

If you're not feeling it, let her know – after the sex has finished. Ask her first what she thought about it, and adjust how you talk about it accordingly.

If she says, "That was fantastic!!" Then you can express your happiness that she loved it, but be open and say what you didn't like about it – maybe that it made you uncomfortable, or that you felt like you were assaulting her, or that it just plain didn't excite you. Then, you can go from there.

If she seems less than enthused about what you've done together, then ask her what would really turn her on. Encourage her to be open with you – after all, you're here to help! Get her to open up about exactly what her fantasy entails, and promise to make it happen the next time.

The most important thing is that she feels safe and comfortable.

You also might feel like you got way too into the domination. If so, you really should take the time to think about why that is so. Perhaps you're feeling a bit underappreciated in the relationship, or you simply don't have enough manly activities in your life that are good outlets for this frame of mind.

However, if you ever get the real urge to cause her pain or to put her down verbally – then stop and seek help.

I'm not saying you're in trouble; it's simply that playing with the dynamics of your relationship might have consequences, and you need to be aware of how it makes you feel when you're participating in a sexual experiment that addresses these dynamics.

You might find during the course of your lovemaking that you fantasize about being this way with another woman. This is completely normal and healthy for a sexually active man. You don't need to feel like you're "cheating" on her or that something is wrong with you because it excites you more to think about this other woman while being with your own woman.

Again, this goes back to the dynamic at play when you're playing with dynamics. Because you are not, I am assuming, a brutish male who stomps all over women's hearts, in essence you are creating a type of role to play while you're fulfilling your partner's alpha male fantasies. And, in the course of playing that role, it might make you feel like a different man. So, it's natural for you to perhaps think about being with a different woman.

Also, it can be hard for a man to be anything less than 100 percent respectful and even deferential to his woman during lovemaking. You might be fantasizing about another woman simply because it may make it easier for you to behave the way you are.

Or, you might just like fantasizing about other women. Again, perfectly normal. Anyone who says they don't is lying.

PART TWO:

FOR WOMEN

BE HONEST. THERE'S SOMETHING MISSING.

What is your husband or boyfriend not doing, but you wish he would?

I'm not talking about the dishes, or dressing better, or chewing with his mouth closed. This book is about how your man does, or does not, satisfy you in the bedroom.

If you're anything like most women out there, you've probably dated a bad boy or two in the past. While you learned soon enough that they're not really long-term boyfriend or husband material, come on, admit it: Your bad boy rocked your world in bed!

He was a total and complete asshole, he never called, he was probably cheating on you, and if he thought about you for five minutes after seeing you it was a big improvement. You're better off without him in your life, I can tell you that!

Once you came to your senses, you found a wonderful man who actually cares about you. You feel for the first time that there is a true partnership, not just dating or a relationship. You're with him for the long haul, and you can't wait to see what the future brings for you both.

The mutual trust, respect and admiration you have for each other are the solid foundation of a strong, healthy and happy relationship. But, what happens when all that love gets in the bedroom? Not much, unfortunately.

Oh, the sex is fine. You feel a connection with him that you'd only read about in books. So much of it feels so right, it's like your bodies were made for each other – two puzzle pieces that together make the whole picture.

But when it comes to the bedroom, sometimes too much respect can be a bad thing. Perhaps you feel a bit of timidity on his part. It can seem like he's afraid to go too far with the passion he so obviously feels for you. Maybe he has balked when you've suggested something a little kinky.

Meanwhile, you feel like you're the one doing all the work, because although he knows your body well and makes you feel great, he's still not touching that part of your sexuality that sends you into the stratosphere.

What your man lacks, and what the bad boys of this world have, use and abuse, is the alpha male touch.

What is an alpha male? He is all man. He knows what he wants, and he's not afraid to get it. He calls the shots. And he knows how to make you feel like a woman. An alpha male is not an asshole, nor does he disrespect women.

The problem is, your man is not going to magically become an alpha male. He's not psychic! And when you have been in a relationship for a while, it can be terribly awkward to suddenly do something drastically different within the boundaries of that relationship.

The good news is, though, that he can be the man you need him to be in the bedroom. He just needs a little direction to get him going. The key is communication – both verbal and non-verbal.

Before you broach this subject, however, you have to know how to define exactly what it is you're looking for. Let's see if we can figure it out together.

Some women want simply to have their men call the shots in bed. They want to feel like the man has the control, because it makes them feel more feminine. There can be something very seductive, and even titillating, about a man who knows exactly what he wants from a woman.

Other women like alpha males in their beds because they want to feel, even if it's just for those moments, like a sexual object. They're tired of proving they're worthy because of their brains or their power plays at work; they want to be worshipped for the goddesses they are!

An even more intense level to which women want to take their desires is that of "rough sex." While this in no way constitutes abuse, there can be some spanking, dirty talk, hair-pulling, clothes torn off or the old slamming-up-against-a-wall-and-having-sex-standing-up situation. They want to feel the hot passion that comes with a man ravishing them.

Another, more psychological motivator behind this desire to be "man-handled," in whatever way is best for you, can come from a need to be absolved of all responsibility for the pleasure you feel.

We women grow up with the phrase, "be a good girl" burned into our brains from a very early age. A lot of times, it's used as an admonishment when we've been acting out.

Then, as we get older, the phrase takes on a whole new meaning – and it's a sexual one. Being a "good girl" can mean dressing a certain way so as not to appear too slutty; not provoking boys, or being too aggressive; waiting to date, or make out, or as we get of age, have sex.

And, now that we are women, this mindset is still reinforced by every possible corner of our society. Even "Sex and The City," for all the talk about liberating the female sexually, still presented sex as something to be giggled over, and many of the ladies' conversations were about the worry of wanting "too much" in bed, or about appearing too slutty.

So, it will come as no surprise that so many women feel that they shouldn't have too much pleasure during sex, or that if they demand what they want it will be misinterpreted in a myriad of ways: that they're slutty, or pushy, or have "a lot" of (i.e. too much) experience. This can be threatening to men, and cause other women to revile them.

We've learned to sit back and take it, so to speak.

Another facet of this same theory is the widely held opinion – no matter how wildly off the mark it is – that women who have been sexually abused or raped were in some way "asking for it," or that they secretly enjoyed it in some way. It's a dark place, psychologically, where no woman wants to go.

We don't want to have that fight in our mind, no matter how delicious it might be at the time, about the struggle between wanting pleasure and wanting to be "a good girl." We feel guilty about going after pleasure, and we feel ashamed after having sought it.

But by "giving in" to an alpha male who controls the sexual agenda within the confines of a healthy relationship, we are liberated from these thoughts and fears. When you are with an alpha male, you feel you have been given permission to show pleasure. After all, it's not your fault – he's the one who's making you get all hot and bothered!

As you can imagine, that can be an uncomfortable responsibility for a man to take on. And, think about how they were raised: be nice to girls, no means no, sexual harassment worries, date rape. Their relationships with women, even non-sexual relationships, have become veritable mine fields of feared missteps or misinterpreted conversations.

So, here you are on the one side with these desires, which come from a complicated place in your heart and mind, and you don't want to talk about these desires for fear of being labeled as something you're not; and on the other side is your man, who loves you and cherishes you and never wants to do you any harm or assert in any way that you are anything less than equal, but who wants to please you sexually.

I'm sure by now you're thinking, "Forget it! That's a conversation I don't want to have. Ever." You're cringing, aren't you, with the thought of how awkward it will be?

Don't worry. I understand that initial reaction, but the truth is that it doesn't have to be awkward, contentious or even all that formal. There are many ways, both verbally and non-verbally, that you can let your partner know that you would like him to be more assertive when it comes to your sexual relationship.

HOW TO LET HIM KNOW WHAT YOU REALLY DESIRE

To get him to the point where he is calling all the shots in the bedroom, you're going to have to do a little bit of calling the shots yourself, even though some of it might seem a bit of a roundabout method.

First, determine for yourself what it is you want. Once you and your partner get into the groove, so to speak, you'll know what feels right and what doesn't, so trust that instinct; but, for starters, you should probably have some idea of what would be too much, or not enough.

You really shouldn't start anything that involves his assertiveness until you fully understand what excites you, why it excites you and what you need for him to do to get you to that point.

For example, do you want him to seem like an authority figure? Do you want to take directions from him, and be told exactly what to do to him, or to yourself, and you simply do what he says?

Or, do you want a bad boy? Do you want someone who smacks your ass, calls you names and does dirty, dirty things to you?

How about a manly-man to flip you around, bend your body in ways you never knew it could, and be put in your place, so to speak.

Then there is always the romantic alpha male – the one who literally whisks you off your feet with no warning, throws you on the bed and makes your every sexual wish come true.

It's really up to you. At this point, you literally only are limited by your imagination. There is nothing off limits. You have to discover exactly what that desire is all about.

Once you know, now you're off to the races. Let's go over some tips for introducing the idea of your man being more assertive in the sex department.

Showing, not telling, is a good way of getting to the point of talking about it, or at least to warm him up to the idea. An awful lot of good stuff can happen in the heat of the moment, and by introducing some rougher elements during your usual lovemaking you can open up the door to more assertiveness, especially if it takes him by surprise.

This can include a variety of actions, which you can do or you can prompt him to do. For example, when you're in the house, grab him, push him toward a wall and pin him there with a long, deep, passionate kiss.

You can start in on some dirty talk, although this doesn't have to be a full dirty conversation – at least at first! You can begin with something as simple as making him say your name. Then you can move onto almost anything that sets you ablaze. It's best if you start the talk, though, and then ask him to respond or to repeat something you've said.

Additionally, it's better if you sound kind of like a porn star when doing this. A bit breathless is good, a little bit of a moan here and there. Lots of "baby" and "making me hot" thrown in there can go a long way.

Then, when he's become comfortable with the level of discourse, shall we say, you want to move into giving direction. If you're doing it doggie-style, you can tell him to spank you. Tell him to hold you down. Tell him to give it to you harder. If a guy thinks he has a good chance of really seeing you explode into ecstasy, he'll take the direction like Pavlov's dog, as long as it's not too far out there at first.

A combination of showing and telling is also good. Say you want him to pull your hair; you can pull on his, then say, "You like that? Yeah? No? That's what I want you to do to me. Pull my hair, yeah, just like that."

Another good tactic to try is to get him really hot and bothered with a lot of teasing and then lie back and say, "Have your way with me" or "Do with me what you will." If you make him hungry enough and then let him have free reign, he'll be all about the alpha maleness at that point.

However, examples like these, at least in the beginning stages, all have to do with you giving direction. And while that can be empowering, in the end, you really want him to take over and be the assertive one who comes up with all these ideas on his own.

The way to make that transition is to talk about what you've already been doing in the bedroom once you've started introducing these more aggressive elements yourself. However, this does not have to be a governmental debriefing! Make it hot, and he'll respond with exactly what you need from him.

THE ALL-IMPORTANT VERBAL CUES

Post-coital conversations are a good place to start talking. Recall the specific things he did to you – even if they were prompted by you – and reinforce how much they turned you on. If you feel like this might be awkward, pretend to yourself that you're describing your favorite parts of your favorite film, or a really delicious part of a wonderful meal you have had.

To further reinforce this, you can send text messages or emails at random times: "Still thinking about that spanking! Yummy!" Or, you can set up a dirty date between the two of you, and say that he can have his way with you tonight. Again, little messages are good for relaying this, as talking it to death is going to make the two of you too self-conscious to be able to enjoy it.

This should all be done and added to gradually so your man doesn't ask what you've done with his woman! Even if he's enjoying the new you, he might want to ask you what's up in a more serious way. After all, one of the signs of a cheating partner is that their sexual tastes change, particularly after a period of lackluster lovemaking between the two of you.

So, you want to be able to explain to him about the changes you've made in the bedroom. There are two important elements to this conversation: that you don't get defensive, and that you don't place the blame at his feet. "Well, you weren't making me happy in the bedroom, so I decided to make some changes" is not the right answer!

Also, a man's ego bruises a lot more easily than you think, which is another reason not to mention any inability on his part.

This doesn't have to be a protracted discussion. It can be as simple as, "It has been making me so hot recently when you're all manly and dominant in the bedroom, I thought we could go further in that direction." Or, you can talk about it in terms of your fantasies of being man-handled, so to speak.

If you want to talk about it in terms of your relationship, you can say, "I love that we're partners in everything we do, but sometimes in the bedroom I want to feel like the weaker sex, you know? I want to feel like a sex object."

Speaking as plainly as this sometimes confuses men! This might be hard to believe, but it's true. This goes back to what we were talking about before, in terms of men being told their whole lives to treat women a certain way, especially when it comes to sex.

Whatever the reason, there are some things you can say to further explain your desires.

If he asks if you want him to get really physical, "No, Honey, but there are times when I want you to call the shots and have your way with me. I might nag you for not cleaning up in the kitchen, but you can be as dirty as you want with me in the bedroom!"

If he asks if you're happy in the relationship, by all means stress as strongly as you can that these desires have no bearing or consequences to your relationship, both day to day and long-term. If possible, try to tie it into a specific thing he did or said that inspired you. "I just got so frisky the other day watching you rebuild the car/play football/chop down that tree, and I was reminded all over again that you are just all man! It turns me on, and I wanted a little bit of that macho lovin' coming my way!"

He can also be confused about the relationship, mistaking your request for something that is lacking in how he treats you. Again, remind him that this pertains to the bedroom only. You love that he treats you with so much respect and that you're seen as an equal partner in the relationship, you just want to feel more like a naughty girl once the bedroom door closes at night.

But, I must emphasize here that too much talk can take all of the fun, passion and spontaneity out of this kind of sexual experimentation. If he keeps asking you to explain or clarify, drag him into the bedroom and show him! Or with a wink, tell him you'll be happy to explain it further, naked, between the sheets – it's up to him to name the time and date.

Once the two of you get into this kind of lovemaking, you want to make sure that the boundaries of your comfort are respected. While this might be a bit rocky at first, some gentle reinforcement and demonstrating can smooth out the way. Again, the heat of the moment is the best time for this, as you'll quickly move onto other more pressing issues!

Sometimes, a simple, "Not so hard, Stud!" can make him pull back or slow down a bit. Other phrases can include, "Not too strong... yes, just like that." "OK, Baby, that's far enough right there." "Now, now, let's not get carried away," said with a cheeky grin and a wink, can soften the criticism.

If you can't help it and an "OUCH!" slips out, take immediate steps to stay in the moment. Chances are that he didn't mean it, and a sexy little one-line joke can bring you both back into the groove.

If he keeps messing up somehow, you don't want him to get performance anxiety. Simply say, "No, Honey, like this" and demonstrate on him, then give a big fat sexy "Oh, yeahhhhh" when he does it right. Men respond really well to positive reinforcement, so don't forget to praise!

If he's a little too into it, switch gears to a slower pace and a more gentle groove. It depends on how freaked out you get about it, but if he seems to have calmed down and it was a one-off, I would stick with the physical reinforcement of slowing it down and making it a softer experience.

However, if you felt like he was out of control, then you need to have a conversation about it; no amount of sexual excitement is worth you feeling unsafe, even for a moment.

The best way is to make it a light conversation: "You were really getting into it, Cowboy. What happened there?" Let him explain, and then finish up with, "Well, just try not to get too scary manly, OK? I still want to see that it's you in there somewhere." If he gets defensive or blames you, calm him down and say that it was fine, but you prefer it to be a bit less than what it was. Then soften the mood with something like, "But don't worry, we'll get the hang of it, just like any new, fun thing!"

For some men who really just don't get it, this behavior might bleed into your daily life. A bit of joking is fun, and a sexy reminder of what you've been up to together. But if he starts to treat you badly at all, or in any way tries to be rough, then it's time to put your foot down and end the shenanigans.

"Hey, wait a minute. That stuff goes on in that room, not out here. Keep it for sexy-time, Bucko." Nice and stern for a moment, and make sure he knows he's out of line.

MAKING IT A FANTASTIC EXPERIENCE FOR BOTH OF YOU

What you need to understand is that there is a powerful psychological dynamic going on, which you created when you introduced this idea. What might seem like fun in the heat of the moment, to either one of you, once replayed in the mind in the light of day can be interpreted any number of ways.

This is what you have to watch out for ... with both of you.

For his part, he might become embarrassed by acting in a way that might seem too different than how he is normally. He might not like himself for acting that way. Is there something wrong with me because I like it too much? Does it mean I am less of a man because I don't like it?

You might feel this too. You might wonder if he's thinking you're a secret slut. You might feel guilty about what you've been doing. Is it wrong to want to feel this way?

Also, despite your assurances, thoughts might creep in, for both of you, about the relationship in general. Is this really because you're not happy in the relationship, and you're just blocking out the reality of the situation?

Whew! Take a breath. It's OK. Let's review a couple of truths:

1. Despite the fact that you've been less than thrilled with what is happening in the bedroom, you are in a loving, committed relationship with a man who cares about you.

2. This is not "wrong." You are two consenting adults who love each other and want to play a bit with your sexual dynamic. This is a perfectly normal urge that happens in the perfectly normal development of a sexual relationship.

3. While it might feel wild for the two of you, on the grand scale of sexual experimentation, kinks and fetishes, it really isn't even remotely freaky. You're simply enhancing the traditional roles of males and females in the bedroom. This is a far cry from,

say, orgies, urination or whipping each other with chains. You're fine.

That said, another truth is that once you get into it with your partner, you might realize it's not nearly as exciting as you had fantasized. Again, this is totally and completely OK! There are any number of perfectly legitimate reasons why this might be the case.

Not all fantasies need to be brought to life in order to be exciting. Some are simply more titillating when they're left in the mind. If this sounds like what you're thinking, it's OK to let the initiative you took kind of go by the wayside in terms of action; you can always fantasize about it on your own time, if you get my drift.

Once you start acting out your fantasies with your partner, it might occur to you that it wasn't your partner you were fantasizing about in the role of alpha male. Again, don't worry about it! It is perfectly healthy to have fantasies featuring men other than your partner. Heck, it's perfectly healthy to have fantasies about women as well!

This might be a bit about the roles involved in what you're doing. You might want to play the role of the innocent girl who's being taken advantage of by a man; maybe it's a 1950s secretary/boss thing; anything is fair game in fantasies. So, it's only natural that while you're playing a certain role in your mind, you are picturing someone else in the other role.

Also, the thought that you're actually doing this together might make some part of you uncomfortable. There are scores of women everywhere who have a hard time being up front about sex and asking for (and receiving) what they want in the bedroom. If this sounds like you, then perhaps fantasizing that someone else is doing all of this is pretty normal.

This also goes back to what we were talking about earlier regarding some women not wanting to take responsibility for their sexual pleasure on a subconscious level. If you feel that someone is making you get this excited by doing something you might consider taboo, then you probably don't want to think that your real-life partner is the person doing it!

WHAT IF IT JUST DOESN'T FEEL RIGHT?

Of course, it might not be as good as you fantasized about simply because it isn't. So, your next question should be, why?

Have you given it enough time? This is an ongoing process, and it might take a good deal of time for you two to "click" when trying out new things in bed, particularly if you've been having the same kind of sex for a long time, or if you haven't been feeling a connection with each other during your lovemaking for a while.

Maybe it's because your desire for male assertiveness isn't sexually based. Perhaps you're reacting to the feeling that you're wearing the pants in this relationship, and you don't love it. If, after taking a good, hard look, this appears to be true, then leave the bedroom antics alone and work on your relationship.

It might not be working because his heart really isn't in it. He might simply not enjoy treating you a certain way, or not derive any pleasure in being dominant in the bedroom. It happens! Perhaps you can talk about it and find something that would be mutually exciting, and get to work on that.

To be blunt, it could be because your guy sucks at it. If you've tried everything you can think of and he's just not getting it, then you have a couple of choices.

For one, you can rent porn and watch it together, showing/telling him how hot certain scenes make you. In this case, porn can literally act as an instruction book! Sometimes, men need to be hit over the head with directions.

If he sucks at it because he's just being too timid, but seems to be into it otherwise, you can show/tell him in bed by really going over the top a few times. You can get a little forceful, say, by making him spank you until it's at the force you want, or by ratcheting up the dirty talk to XXX level.

But, if he really just plain sucks at it, it's OK to drop it and go back to sexy alone time with your fantasies. Again, now that he's at least open to experimentation, you can find something that pleases you both, perhaps with something of the same kinds of elements involved, which would bring him to that point from another direction.

The thing I really do want to stress, though, is that you make sure that this is only about sexual experimentation and not about your relationship outside the bedroom. I bring this up again because sometimes it can be so hard to separate the two.

For example, there is the phrase "make-up sex" for a reason. Sometimes, sex after an argument can be a healer, or it seals a new agreement or compromise made by the two of you. There is a powerful psychological connection between you during this kind of sex, and chances are your man is more assertive than ever during make-up sex.

Therefore, you might try to get a rise out of him, as it were, by picking a fight with him that you know will lead to make-up sex, whether it's just so you can feel that assertion coming through, or as a way to tell him afterward that that is the kind of sex you're talking about.

I implore you to fight this urge. Angry sex, or make-up sex, or any sex that comes out of an emotional state of mind from non-sexual events, will only serve to hurt both of you in the end. This is simply not the way to go about doing it, no matter how hot it is as it is happening.

However, the dynamic might swing the other way, too. Maybe you and your partner had great sex in the beginning of your relationship. Often, a man will be more assertive during sex as a way to claim you as his own, or to impress you, or any variety of reasons. Or, it could just have been that the two of you were more adventurous in the beginning, as you pushed the boundaries and got to know each other's bodies and sexual preferences.

But, as you became an item, committed to each other and relaxed into your lives together, so too did your sex life relax. It's perfectly normal, and livening up the proceedings with a bit of sexual experimentation can be just the ticket to put the spark back into your relationship.

The problem, though, might not be with your sexual relationship; it might be with your relationship as a whole. And instead of asking yourself the tough questions about your current situation and how it might affect your future, you prefer to channel your unhappiness with him as a life partner into "fixing" him as a sexual partner.

Again, anytime you try to fix the relationship by fixing the sex, it's going to become glaringly obvious that your efforts are misguided. Work on the relationship and let a better sex life come as a result.

In other words, you might have discovered you're with a man who really has no alpha male tendencies to speak of in any aspect of his life, and you have to decide whether or not that's a problem for you.

PART THREE:

TIPS AND SUGGESTIONS FOR **COUPLES**

COMING TOGETHER...TO MAKE THINGS HAPPEN

Now we're ready to talk about the good stuff! But, before we get rolling here, I would like to reiterate some important points we went over in the advice for women and the advice for men sections of this book. It's really important to understand the basics, and this also will serve as a primer for you bad boys and girls who skipped ahead!

A woman wanting her man to be more assertive or dominant in the bedroom is not a reflection on the relationship at all. While experimenting with alpha male tactics during sex might put a spark into your relationship, all in all this is simply about what goes on between the sheets.

If either of you have read this book and your thoughts keep drifting back to instances in your day-to-day relationship where this advice would come in handy, then stop here and work on your relationship. You can come back to this book once your relationship is back to being a healthy and happy one.

Similarly, this advice is not for new couples or for casual sexual encounters. There needs to be a trusting bond between you, and that comes with time and experience with each other. There is a lot of communication necessary to make this a successful sexual endeavor; anything less and you risk being misunderstood at a crucial time.

Another thing this book **is NOT about is BDSM techniques**. That stands for Bondage/Domination/Sadism/Masochism, and we're talking about a whole other ball of wax – in some ways, literally. If you're looking for more hard-core sex advice, this might serve as an excellent albeit extremely introductory guide to the power dynamic behind BDSM. But, this has nothing to do with that world at all. If you are interested in BDSM, then I encourage you to do some lengthy research before even thinking about engaging in it. It's not just all whips and chains.

A Word To the Women:

Remember, make sure you have a clearly defined idea of what you want from your man when you say you want him to be more assertive in the bedroom. This will help you define boundaries later on.

Also, keep in mind that at no time do you have to continue with this type of sex play. We'll talk about this more in a bit, but for now, be aware that just because you brought it up doesn't mean you have to see it through. If you are ever uncomfortable, or if it just plain isn't doing it for you, then stop.

To get your man to alpha male status, you're going to have to give him some direction and there might have to be some strange conversations about what you want. Keep in mind that your man loves you and wants you to be happy! And, once he gets the hang of it, it's going to be fun for him too!

Make sure your man understands that this is not a reflection of his masculinity at all. This is a sexual desire YOU have, that HE can fulfill.

A Word To the Men:

Guys, I understand this might be a new and strange thing for you, so I'd like to remind you of a few things as we move on to the down and dirty techniques of being more sexually dominant.

As we told the ladies above, and as your own lady should be telling you, just because she wants you to be more assertive in the bedroom does not mean she thinks you're a girly-man; nor does it mean she wants you to beat her.

Your role in this endeavor is to LISTEN to what she is telling you, and to make a concerted effort to be on her same wavelength once you two start getting busy. She'll let you know what she wants; she'll let you know when what you're doing isn't working; and she probably won't need to tell you when it IS working, if you get my meaning.

Safe Words:

While I have stressed above that male assertiveness in the bedroom has nothing to do with the BDSM culture, we are going to take a page from their book, just to be extra cautious.

We're going to talk about safe words.

Safe words are traditionally used in instances when there is a level of pain involved in the sex play, or if the situation requires, as part of the scenario, that one or the other partner says, "No" or "Stop" but is not supposed to mean it.

We're going to get into some of the more intense games the two of you can play at a point later in the book, but anytime you are dealing with the male/female power dynamic, it's better to be safe than sorry.

Simply put, a safe word is one that, when said by either partner, the action immediately stops. You should agree on what word it is, and it should be the same word for both of you. It also should have absolutely nothing to do with sex or any kind of scenario you're playing out.

Common safe words are color names, city names or state names. Choose just one word, not a phrase; and make sure it's easy to remember!

If you're ever in a situation where the safe word is spoken – again, by either of you – and you've stopped immediately, don't break apart or hop out of bed and get dressed. It takes courage to say a safe word, and most likely it will leave both of you feeling vulnerable.

So, make sure to hug, cuddle, lie together and be very gentle with one another after it's been spoken. This is not a time for blame, or an argument, or stony silence. Let the moment pass, get to a mental place where you both feel calm and secure, and then you can talk about what happened, and how it can be changed or avoided next time around.

The next time you have sex, it should be in a more "traditional" style, and it should be more about lovemaking than about any kind of experimentation or anything rough and tumble. Then you can work your way back up to whatever you want to do.

LET'S START OUT WITH SOME DIRTY TALK

Before the two of you get down to business, a bit of dirty talk might be just the ticket to get you on the same wavelength. It's also a good way to set the boundaries of your assertive sex play without having to stop what either of you are doing physically. And talking dirty is fun!

While it might be uncomfortable at first, there are real benefits to talking dirty where sexual experimentation is concerned. For one, as I've just said, it helps set boundaries without the physical aspect. By being able to go over the top in words, you won't have to go there in deed.

For example, let's say you're having phone sex. You're getting each other all hot and bothered, and then he suggests something that's way over the top, say, slapping her face when she's said something about being especially naughty.

Now, there is a chance she might love it, but there is a chance she really, really won't love it. If he were to take that chance physically, it could get ugly. But by taking that chance in words only, he's giving her the opportunity to say, "Yes, Baby, slap me again" or "Oh no, Baby, be gentle with your little bitch" or whatever you've got going on. No harm, no foul. You've both learned something, and you can move on without any recriminations.

During sex, dirty talk can also make things more exciting without actually having to "go there." The two of you could be having totally normal, traditional, "boring" sex, but by talking a blue streak about fantastic circumstances or some different roles that really turn you on, you're transporting yourselves to places you might not be able to go in reality.

For our purposes – that is, in getting the male partner to be more assertive, more alpha male, more in control of what's going on in that bedroom of yours – the woman should be the one to start the ball rolling. It's going to be her way of saying what she wants, without making it sound like a complaint or a laundry list!

And guys, it's your job to listen closely and follow her lead, at least at first. Then, once you have a better idea of what she's into and not so into, you can really start to pick up that ball and run with it. You can test the boundaries of your alpha male kingdom without perhaps embarrassing yourself, or without being worried about taking it too far or not far enough.

For many couples, dirty talk has changed their sex lives for the better. However, dirty talk isn't already in some couples' sexual repertoire. And that's totally OK! But understand, it could feel super awkward when you're getting started if you're not "in the moment" together, or sometimes it can just plain sound silly as hell.

If you're one of these couples, then I can recommend a few things to help you get started.

First, try not talking at all; try writing. It can be easier to take yourself to naughty land if you don't have to hear your own voice saying things. We'll go over sexy scribbles in a moment, but there is one warning here: other people can read your writing as well! So be careful not to embarrass yourself or your partner by being reckless with your words.

- If you are in the habit of talking with instant messenger, start a provocative conversation on chat.
- Send text messages to each other's cell phones with vivid descriptions of what you want to do to each other.
- If you communicate by email on personal accounts (as opposed to work-based addresses), write out your fantasies, or team up to write a continuing dirty story by sending it back and forth to each other.
- Mad Libs is a word game in which the answers to word prompts you're given are revealed as part of a story. Go to a sex novelty shop and pick up a dirty Mad Libs, then play it together! They can be fun and silly, and very, very naughty.
- Send a greeting card in the mail with salacious salutations, or perhaps an explicit invitation.

Once you have established that each of you can hold your own in a dirty conversation, it's time to move on to talking dirty. However, even this can be accomplished without being face to face, at least when you're starting out.

Do either one of you go on business trips? Try having long-distance phone sex. This works best when the entire conversation revolves around sex; don't start out by reminding him to take out the trash, or letting her know that package she was waiting for arrived. You can have that conversation in its own phone call.

Phone sex in this instance is a good way to get the man in control. He can direct his partner to do things, like undressing, touching herself, etc. He can gain the upper hand without the possibility of being intimidated by having her there in front of him.

And for her part, this is the time to really experiment with pushing the limits of his masculine side. Go over the top, really let him know that he is all man and he can have his way with you.

So, while there are times that he will be calling the shots during phone sex, there should also be times when she is the one talking about her fantasies in explicit detail. Let yourselves get excited, and let your partner know that what's happening is exciting you.

Another fun, sexy phone game is to leave each other voicemail messages. (Again, please be mindful of your partner's habits; if they prefer to listen to their voice mail on speaker, you should probably avoid this game.) And remember, leave the messages to pick up milk on the way home to a separate call.

You might just want to let your partner know exactly what's going through your mind. Or, you can leave a detailed treasure hunt of a message, or inform them of what they'll find when they get home. Here are some examples. (And, you probably don't have to say who it is; I suspect they'll figure it out soon enough.)

- Ladies, these voicemails can be invitations, directions or simply your fantasies. Tell him that you'll be in the bedroom when he gets home, naked and waiting for him to have his way with you. Describe to him a particularly exciting moment from the last time you had sex – in graphic detail – or do the same describing something you want him to do to you. This reinforces the stuff you like while turning him on! Or, you can start a game, perhaps asking him to give you a specific instruction that you'll have to follow the next time you're having sex.

- Guys, this is your chance to start the game of assertiveness without having the worry of performance anxiety. You can get her so hot that by the time you are both in the bedroom, you are home free! Leave her a detailed message explaining exactly what you're going to do to her body when you both get home tonight. Or, tell her you have an entire evening planned; have her go home, put on a specific outfit you love, and be ready to go out at a certain time. Perhaps remind her of a certain moment from the night before, and tell her you're going to do that and more the next time.

And, hey, if they pick up the phone instead, don't chicken out! Simply say, "Hi, I wanted to tell you that ..." deliver your message without stopping, then hang up. Who wouldn't love a phone call like that?

Now, let's talk dirty while you're face to face.

If you're not used to being chatty in between the sheets but you've started talking dirty outside the bedroom, bringing up those "heated" discussions while getting your groove on can make for a good transition.

If you've had phone sex, for example, you can start out by having each other reenact some of the things you did to yourselves, or "did" to each other (i.e., what you described doing to each other). Again, this is something the woman can bring up at first, but really the man should be taking the ball and running with it after some prompting.

For example, a good way to direct her actions is to tell her that it turned him on so much when she was describing, say, how she was touching herself during a particular call. Have her reenact it while you watch, then you can join in.

Or, she can say how it made her feel when he was talking about doing this or that to her, and that she's fantasized about finally being able to have him do it now. Then, he can include the sexy talk while he's doing it: "Which part did you love, Baby? Was it when I said I was going to do this?" (Do it.) "Or was it when I talked about doing this (do it) until I made you come?"

As I've said before, dirty talk can also be a good start when he is a bit shy about actually physically asserting himself with her. He can maybe thrust a bit harder, a bit faster, but talk about more advanced moves: "Is this what you want, Baby? You want a real man? I'll show you who's a real man, yeah. I'm giving it to you hard and fast. You like that? You want me to get rough with you, huh? Oh, I'll do all that and more, is that what you want, Baby?"

Then, of course, the dirtier talk can be used as an assertive technique all on its own. This will require a bit of trial and error, and maybe a conversation or two out of bed, before he finds the right words that make her go over the edge into oblivion.

For example, if she likes to be made to feel like a sexual object, he can accommodate that desire by talking about her body in the most objectified terms as possible. The key to this is to be raunchy and dirty, while praising her – NOT to put her down, offend or insult her!

That is unless she specifically asks for that. She might want you to call her a whore, a slut, a bitch, Daddy's little bitch, nothing but a vessel for your seed, etc. But that has to be a specific direction from her, or else you might get slapped. Go ahead and ask her what she's comfortable hearing from you.

Otherwise, talking dirty in this instance is just that – describing what you are doing, or what you love about her, or what you want from her in the most graphic, raunchy language you can think of. Some examples would be:

- "Take that dress off and let me see those luscious tits of yours."

- "Turn over, I'm going to give you my cock from behind, and you're going to feel every inch of it."
- "You like it when I slap your juicy ass?" (Slap) "You want me to do it again?" (Slap) "You want a spanking, my bad girl?" (Slap, slap, slap)

You get the idea. If you need inspiration or want to get the lingo right, watch porn films, read *Penthouse Letters* or listen to really raunchy rap music.

And as for the ladies, dirty talk is a powerful communication tool to guide your man through your desires, and to let him know if he's gone too far, as well. Dirty talk allows you to do all this without breaking the mood.

For example, if you want him to be more aggressive, goad him into taking it to the next level. "I know you've got more to show me, come on, Baby, give it to me. Show me what a man you are, put me in my place. Is that the best you've got? Come on, I want it rough, baby."

If you want him to talk dirty to you, start it yourself. "Am I your little slut? Yeah? Tell me I'm just your little whore." "Tell me who's the man. Are you the man?" "Can you feel how wet I am, Baby? That's because you turn me on when you take control. Tell me how good it feels."

And for those times that he might go too far, you can smooth things over easily and move on. "Ooh, Baby, not so rough, OK? Just like that, yeah." "Ow, that one hurt baby, don't be so rough with your little lady." The key to this is to keep the dirty talk up with praise as soon as he's adjusted his behavior. "Yeah, that's the way I like it, Sugar, just like that."

Of all the tricks, tips and techniques we talk about in this book, talking dirty is probably the most useful for couples who are experimenting with male assertiveness. It's a mode of communication that is unlike any other! A tremendous amount of information can be given with a bare minimum of words, and in a language unique to the two of you.

So, don't be afraid to talk dirty!

Just a final thought on the matter, though: try your best to respect the dirty talk your partner gives. Don't laugh at the terms they use, or make fun of them later on about something they might have said in the heat of the moment. As I'm sure you can tell from reading this section, dirty talk can look pretty silly written down, and it can be just as silly taken out of context. Play nice, you two!

ASSERTIVE ORAL PLEASURE

Now that we have covered talking dirty to help along the alpha male, we can incorporate what we've learned into the next step of this sexual experiment: assertive oral pleasure.

But before we get into the one-on-one game of oral sex, I'd like to back up for a moment and talk about how this can be preceded with some masturbation "games" that can be an exciting way to have him assert his authority over the proceedings.

Dirty talk is an integral part of this section, both with masturbation and oral sex. However, the level of verbal domination you want to take it to is entirely up to the two of you, as well as how comfortable you feel saying raunchy things and how much pleasure she gets from being verbally directed to do things (as opposed to physical direction or manipulation).

That being said, let's get started! There are two ways assertive action during masturbation can be handled.

The first is having her masturbate while he gives her specific direction. This can start with telling her to undress, and can be as specific as telling her which pieces of clothing to take off in a certain order. Or, he can wait until she is in position. Again, that position can be dictated by him as well.

Then, he tells her where to touch, how to touch, and whether to go slower or faster. Again, this can be explicit, in both meanings of the word; he can tell her exactly what to do, and he can also use raunchy language.

It all depends on what part of the alpha male personality is most exciting to her. If she gets off on being completely dominated by him, then he should give exact instructions. If it's the fact that she's doing this for his pleasure, then more general directions are better; she might get too distracted by being told exactly what to do.

Creativity can come into play. He doesn't have to give her direction, he can talk about him doing these things to her: "Now I'm touching your left breast, I'm caressing it ..."

He can also get into the act, with a show-and-tell kind of game. For every move he wants her to make, he does it to her first, and then lets her do it after.

It can also be a tease-and-denial scenario, where he watches her bring herself to the brink of orgasm and then tells her to stop, then begin again, over and over again.

He can join in, masturbating as he becomes aroused by what she's doing; then the two of you can come together. Or, he can wait until she's really into it, and then "take over" from there, either by fingering her to orgasm, performing oral sex on her or having intercourse. Or, he can wait until she has an orgasm, and then go to town on her in any way he sees fit!

Turning the tables a bit, the other way is that he can have his masturbation be the focal point of the scenario. He might have her do a strip tease, dance or perform other activities (move into certain positions, or put on makeup or brush her hair, or anything else that is feminine for her and turns him on) while he watches and masturbates. He tells her what to do, and she complies.

Again, this can end any number of ways, from mutual masturbation, to her taking over for him, to oral sex, to intercourse. And, as always, dirty talk rules!

As far as oral sex goes, there are pretty much two ways for this as well, with variations on each theme.

For Her:

Normally, a man giving oral pleasure to a woman is viewed as a submissive act on his part. However, men honestly enjoy a good munching, and there should be no reason why this cannot be seen as him exercising his right to pleasure through pleasuring her.

Aggressively eating her out involves lots of fun things: he can grab a hold of her ass, hard, and squeeze; in the same position, use that grabbing as a way to guide her hip movements and rhythm; reaching for the breasts, with some rougher handling or nipple pinching; grabbing her thighs; biting her thighs; aggressive finger thrusting inside her, with an increasing number of fingers; the same for her ass; and quickly transitioning from eating her out to thrusting himself hard inside her.

Also, he can have her on her hands and knees and eat her out from behind. This is a good position if he wants to transition into intercourse; also, he can more easily grab a hold of her and dictate her hip movements and rhythms while he's at it.

Another nifty little assertive trick here is to reach up and insert a finger or two into her mouth - particularly if you have used it in her vagina already (no ass-to-mouth!). This is a more subtle form of penetration, but still sends the same message.

The general feeling, though, is that this is for his pleasure, and he is dominating her; it's not to be viewed as him worshipping her, as more submissive, gentle oral sex would be. This can be a good scenario to experiment with when the man is still a bit timid about really asserting himself. At no time, though, should she do any face-sitting. This is all about the man, remember?

For Him:

A woman giving a man a blowjob is perhaps one of the most submissive acts in a traditional lovemaking repertoire. So, it can lend itself to all kinds of nasty fun in the alpha male sexual scenarios, too.

However, there are so many men who are keenly aware of the power dynamic at play; even if these men are into the whole idea of male domination in the bedroom, they can get uncharacteristically shy when it comes to blowjobs.

Also, guys have learned early on that doing anything to upset a girl leads to no more blowjobs, so they've gotten very, very careful about doing anything that might highlight the submissive aspects of it.

Well, guys, now is your chance to get it all out of your system, because if she really wants you to be more aggressive sexually, the blowjob is the place where her desires will be put to the test!

However, it's also the place where you're most likely to go overboard. So, it's important to talk to each other about her comfort zone. If you feel this might be an awkward conversation, remember, it won't be nearly as awkward as the result of her aggression while your penis is in her mouth. One word: *OUCH.*

All that being said, there are a few ways to approach the blowjob from the alpha male perspective. I'll say it again, though: it really needs to be thought about and agreed upon beforehand.

The first is the blowjob-on-demand. Unlike what I had mentioned a while back, this is the equivalent of "Bitch, make me a sandwich." With prior agreement from her, he can feel free to make her blow him any old time it pleases him.

Another tactic is to give her the order during foreplay. This is particularly powerful if he has worked her into quite a lather first. It's a sign of, hey, my pleasure comes first (no pun intended).

Yet another time is during intercourse, after she has come. Making her taste her own juices is an aggressive action. (Obvious note here: this is not to be done if there has been any anal sex!)

No matter when or how you choose to approach the blowjob, dirty talk is a huge part of it. Again, this should be something agreed upon by the both of you. She's already being submissive by giving the blowjob, and that has been amplified by the fact that he has instructed her to do it. Some girls will get an extra kick out of the man ratcheting up the submission angle; others will draw the line and blowjobs on demand, and leave it at that.

Another point here is that there are physical possibilities when wanting to highlight the assertiveness aspect of the blowjob. Let me beat a dead horse here and say that yes, again, this is something that should be worked out beforehand.

He can force her head down onto his penis. Using both hands, he can dictate the rhythm. He can pull her hair back to be able to see better, or simply pull it to show his pleasure. He can stand, or sit on the edge of the bed, and make her kneel in front of him.

In a particularly aggressive move, he can have her on her back, and thrust into her mouth. This is good for switching it up with tit-fucking, if that is something that floats your boats. Be careful with the gag reflex in this position, however.

He can also ask that she dress a certain way, or be completely naked, or just wear sexy heels, or whatever makes it more about his pleasure.

PLEASURABLE, ROUGH INTERCOURSE

Yes! Now we're talking. Enough with the foreplay; let's get into the action! In this section, we'll talk about all the ways men can be more assertive while having sex. Finally!

Just a note for those of you who skipped directly to this section: *don't*. Go back and read the entire book. There is a lot going on when this powerful male-female dynamic is exercised, and if you don't understand it all, someone's going to get hurt. Maybe not physically, but definitely emotionally. Please be smart, communicate, and make sure your relationship outside the bedroom is healthy, happy and solid as a rock.

OK, OK, I've lectured enough. Let's get it on.

Assertive Positions

Obviously, having the woman be on top is not the height of male assertiveness. If she's riding him like a cowgirl, it has become all about her, and that's not what we're talking about here, are we?

However, there are some ways to assert authority while the woman is in this position. For starters, he should be grabbing onto her hips, and making her match her movements to his own. He should be dictating the rhythm; if she tries to change it, his grasp should get stronger.

Also in this position, rough breast play is a good assertive action. Or, have her come down to him, and suck, twist and nibble on her breasts.

By incorporating dirty talk into this position, however, she can be left to her own devices, so to speak, while he talks about how much of a slut she is for taking pleasure in it, how much she loves to ride that big hard cock, etc.

Just as obviously, however, the man being on top is by far the more aggressive stance when having sex. But this position, called the Missionary position, has been the death of so many relationships ... death by sexual boredom. So, let's talk about how to roughen it up around the edges a bit, and make it be all about the alpha male conquering his woman.

The Missionary position can be manipulated in a variety of ways that shows her who's boss. They include:

Her legs up over his shoulders; him kneeling up a little and thrusting in hard. This is also a good position for spanking while in the Missionary position.

- Pushing her legs to their widest position, again with the man kneeling.

"Balls-deep" is the phrase you're looking for here.

- Forcing her to bend her legs to her chest, so her knees are by her ears, and putting his weight on her. Done correctly, he might be able to have both hands free to grab her hips for rhythm control, or for some spanking.
- Pinning her hands down beside or above her head. By using both hands to do so, she is effectively pinned down; by using one hand, he can hold hers down while using his other hand to have his way with her while he's inside her: grabbing a breast, tweaking a nipple, a finger or fingers or thumb in her mouth, tickling her clitoris, etc.
- Lifting her toward him, and pulling her head back by her hair so he can nibble on her throat.

Doggie-style sex is great for the alpha male. He has much more control over her in this position.

- He can grab a hold of her hips to dictate rhythm and movement. Also, he can be in control of how hard and deep he thrusts into her.

- There can be lots of slapping and spanking in this position.
- He can lean over and play with her breasts, or reach around to play with her clitoris.
- He can cup his hand around her cheek, and force a finger into her mouth for sucking.
- There can be a bit of ass play here, whether using fingering or applying pressure. (Just be mindful of where that finger goes next.)

While other positions can be pleasurable for you both, these are the only two where real domination can be asserted. However, this is about the bedroom only; why don't we move on to the rest of the house, and see what we can find?

Gauge your own alpha male levels, and see if you can coordinate those times you're feeling like the king of the world with getting it on with your honey. For example, are you feeling testosterone-y after a pickup basketball game with the guys or a hard workout? Let her experience your sweaty, manly self and your finely toned muscles.

Or, how about that morning wood? Put it to good use and ravish her! Now, that's the way to start a day.

Depending on the level of comfort and your respective heights, there are many places in the home where some quick-and-dirty, rough sex can be had.

The keys to having successful alpha male sex in other areas of the home are spontaneity and roughness. When a man wants his woman, he doesn't care where they are or what they are doing, he's going to take her and have his way with her.

- Bend her over the sofa armrest and "do" her from behind. The same goes for the kitchen counter and dining room table.
- Home office? Swipe off the papers from the desk, and throw her on top of it.
- Watching TV? How about she blows him during the commercial break, or he spreads her out on the coffee table.
- Give her a good pounding while she's sitting on the washing machine.
- If she's going up the stairs in front of you, wait until she is almost at the top, then lean her over so she's on the landing, and kneel behind her.

- Push her against a wall, pin her there and have sex standing up. Lift her up so she wraps her legs around you.
- Is she having a nice, hot, steamy shower? Well, what are you waiting for? Get in there!

With this kind of inspiration in mind, you two might start to see your house in a whole new way. You're really only limited by your imagination! Remember, make it quick and dirty.

And ladies, you can give your man a little nudge in this direction. Walk up those steps in a short skirt with no panties on. Lean over seductively to get the dishes out of the dishwasher. Hop up on the kitchen counter with your legs spread while you're having a chat. He'll get the message soon enough!

Anal Sex

Anal sex really is the final frontier for alpha male sex. However, it's really not something you want to tackle for the first time while experimenting with sexual assertiveness. This is because it needs to be introduced slowly, not only in a gradual way into your sexual repertoire, but also physically slowly when you're actually doing it.

There are some non-negotiable rules about anal:

1. Use lubrication, and by that, I mean go into a store and buy real lube. Not spit, not olive oil, not massage oil. LUBE.
2. Never go ass-to-mouth. No blowjobs after anal sex, no kissing after rimming, no eating her out after rimming her.
3. Never go ass-to-vagina. Once you're in, you're in to win.

Any action near the anus should first be done with your fingers. Start by caressing lightly – like, butterfly-kisses-lightly – her ass cheeks and the crack of her ass. Keep moving back to fingering her vaginal area. Then, massage her ass using a bit more pressure, pushing with your palm a bit along her ass crack. While fingering her, move further and further back toward her anus, but don't enter. Finally, work up to fingering the outside of her anus.

When it comes time to penetrating her anus with your finger, there are a few things to remember:

1. Make sure she is physically relaxed and in a comfortable position before you try it.
2. Have some lube nearby. You don't want to be going in there dry.
3. Make sure your nails are clipped short and smooth, with no hangnails or jagged edges.
4. You can't go back to fingering her vaginal area, so make sure she's either already had an orgasm or that you're willing to completely switch up your sexual position.

Gradually increase the pressure of your finger a bit at a time. Once finger penetration has been established, entering with two fingers should be done at the same time. Don't get one in there and then try to squeeze the other one in; you run the risk of tearing sensitive skin.

While keeping an ever-steady rhythm, move your body lengthwise alongside hers, with yourself partly on top of her, and using your rhythmic movements, get both of your bodies into the rhythm of lovemaking.

When it's penis time, you'll want to do a little finger play at first, and get her comfortable. Let the tip of your penis push against her anus for several rounds of rhythmic movements, and slowly ease it in. Slow rhythm, slow penetration. It will take you a while to get fully inside her, and let yourself just kind of be in there a while before you start going for the gold.

And don't forget, no matter how flaccid you become after orgasm, come out just as slowly as you went in. Don't forget to check and make sure the condom came out with you.

The very act of anal sex is so dominant on the part of the male, that there really is no reason to cowboy it up while you're back there. However, again, this is something that should be discussed between the two of you. If she winds up loving it and is totally into it, feel free to experiment with rough sex through the back door.

"Rough" Techniques

We've talked about several positions so far, and several different kinds of sex, including mutual masturbation and oral sex. Now, we're going to delve a bit deeper into the techniques that can make these activities become all about the alpha male. We've gone over some of them before, but in this section I'll explain them in a bit more detail, so it's clear to both of you what is involved (although I'll be speaking to the guys here).

Physical Assertion

Slapping and spanking are different from each other, believe it or not. Spanking is harder, for one, and is only done on her ass. Slapping is a bit lighter, and depending on the agreement you both come to, can be done on the ass, the outer thighs, and for the more advanced, and rarely, the face.

With any hitting like that, though, especially in sensitive areas, you want to gently rub first, then slap, then gently rub again. Otherwise, there can be an abusive connotation that you really don't want lingering in the air. Also, it gives her warning that you're about to do it, and afterward you're doing for her what everyone's natural reaction is to a physical action like that – gently rubbing the area to soothe it.

Hair pulling should not be done from the ends of the hair; that HURTS, and not in a good way. Instead, work your hand into her hair, as if you were going to cradle her head, and pull from the roots. This gives you greater control over her head movements, and will not hurt nearly as much.

Grabbing and clutching are excellent assertive actions to take, and they can help you communicate your passion and your level of excitement, too. As we've already learned, grabbing her hips or torso can help you control rhythm and movement. But sometimes, it's just great to hang on for the ride!

You can also clutch her thighs, her upper arms, or any part of her that gives you the dominating position. How much force with which you do this, again, is entirely up to the both of you.

Pinching and tweaking her breasts, nipples or ass can be extremely titillating for her. There is a bit of the pleasure/pain principle involved here, and if your girl is into it, go for it.

Nibbling and biting can be a fun, primal way to show you're the alpha male. Just be careful about breaking skin and leaving marks in obvious places!

Throwing her onto the bed is fun, dominant and oh-so-caveman. Just lift her up, extend your arms and let go. She'll bounce around once or twice, and then it's time for you to get on top, Baby!

We've talked about pushing her up against a wall a bit, but let me tell you that this is something you should seriously consider. Women who are into alpha males LOVE this. The only thing you need to remember is that this is in fact a combination of pushing her, and pushing against her, so that you follow her. Otherwise, you're just slamming her around, and that's not fun for anyone. Your best bet is to start kissing her away from the wall – strongly, passionately – run your hands down from her shoulders to her upper arms, then grab a hold of her and using your body, push her against the wall and press up against her.

For an added thrill, you can continue to run your hands down to her wrists, then move her hands up the wall and pin her there.

Which leads me to the next physical trick: pinning her down. When she lacks the ability to grab at you, you've gained total control. Just remember to do it for short bursts; you don't want her to panic.

Sexual Assertion

Any anal penetration, even with your finger, is an aggressive move. It's best done while you're pleasuring her in other ways, unless you want to dedicate an entire session to anal; in that case, do whatever works best for the two of you.

Going from doggie-style to anal sex can be a way to take it to the next level; just remember to make sure she is relaxed, don't go in with only one thrust, and don't go back to vaginal sex.

Making her kiss you after you've gone down on her, or having her give you a blow-job after you've been inside her, are two huge alpha male tactics.

Delaying her orgasm is another powerful way to show her you're in charge. Simply get her beyond excited and then stop. Do it over and over again until she is begging you to let her have an orgasm. Even then, let it go one or two more rounds.

Assertion Through Orgasm

Anytime you do something unexpected with your own orgasm, you are demonstrating your control over the situation. Here are some ways to dominate her with semen.

While you're in the doggie-style position, pull out and come onto her back, either by masturbating or pushing against her ass. For an added touch, massage your semen into her back.

While in the Missionary position, you can pull out and masturbate to orgasm, coming on her pubic hair, her torso, her breasts or even her face. Or, you can straddle her and masturbate to the same effect.

These are two pretty intense examples of male dominance; they really should be tried only after you've been experimenting for a bit. Also, once the sex is over you can reinforce the fact that you know it's a fantasy by helping her clean off your semen, or in the case of it being on her back, clean it up for her. Make sure to do this very gently, and give her a little cuddle afterward.

Whatever you do, don't just leave her there with your semen all over her unless she has explicitly stated that that is what she wants you to do. Some women like their alpha male fantasy to extend to the moments after the sex has finished, as well, and that's totally normal. But otherwise, leaving her there takes you from alpha male to asshole in one giant step.

HEIGHTEN THE INTENSITY WITH TOYS AND GAMES

Once you have established this alpha male element to your lovemaking, you can get to a point where the experimentation can be taken to a whole new level. In this section, we're going to talk about new things you can introduce into your repertoire that can keep things spicy and feeling new and exciting.

Toys

Dildos and vibrators can offer you multiple options for penetrative fun. With a vibrator, there can be lengthy orgasm teasing/denial sessions, for example. There are small vibrators available that can be run over the entire body for extra "tortures" of pleasure.

Combined with dirty talk, he can describe what he's doing to her and how he feels while he's penetrating her with a dildo or vibrator. This allows him total control. He is not monitoring his own sexual activity as well, so he can concentrate better, while giving her intense pleasure.

Dildos can be used during oral sex to accompany what he's doing with his mouth. During intercourse, there can be anal and vaginal action for maximum penetration.

These devices can also be used while he's making her masturbate, particularly if he has her describe what he's doing to her while she's using them. For an added twist, perhaps while she's away on business, he can have her masturbate while fantasizing about what he'd be doing to her, and then give him a hand job upon her return while she tells him about it.

Of course, household objects can be used as well; wine bottles, the TV remote, carrots and cucumbers can all be converted to instant playthings when the passion strikes! Just make sure they're clean before inserting into any sensitive areas.

While I don't want to get into a whole discussion about bondage - as I've said before, this is not that kind of book - he can use soft items, like scarves or neckties, to tie her wrists while he goes to town on her body. There can be lengthy teasing sessions, and it can allow him to be a bit gentler to offset the harshness of being bound.

However, this is an activity that is on a more advanced level, and there should be clear boundaries and a time limit agreed upon before the games begin.

If you would like to achieve the intensity of slapping or spanking but the thought of actually doing it makes either one of you uncomfortable, then other, more playful options can be explored. You could use a paper fan, or a linen napkin, or even a dishtowel for the same effect without any bruising or panic.

Blindfolding – again, with a scarf or other soft material – can lend a whole new experience to your lovemaking, and puts the man squarely in the driver's seat. While she is blindfolded, tease her until she can't take it anymore! Be as quiet as you can, and don't let on where you're going to touch her next.

Games

Role-playing in a sexual context is an entire fetish in and of itself; again, this book is not about that, but I'd like to show you how you can incorporate it into your alpha male scenarios for a bit of fun. Role-playing can also be a great way to break the ice, and can allow each partner to become more involved in the scenario than if they were simply "being themselves."

Basically, any alpha male/submissive female combination that excites you both is fair game for role-playing. You can have a successful scenario simply choosing roles and talking through them (dirty talk, of course); or you can go whole hog and get costumes and props! It really depends on your comfort level and what makes the alpha male dynamic come more alive for you.

Some popular combinations include:

- Professor and student
- Football star and cheerleader or fan
- Boss and secretary
- Doctor and nurse
- Doctor and patient
- Rich man and poor girl
- Rough trade and rich girl
- Client and hooker or escort
- Handyman or deliveryman and housewife
- Experienced man and virgin

But really, it's any combination that floats your boat!

There is an even more intense "game" that can be played, although I would advise it only if both of you are completely honest and in 100 percent agreement about the alpha male scenario. It's a rape fantasy, and while it's a very real fetish in the sexual community, rape is also a very real, and very terrible crime about power and control. Proceed with caution.

There is no negotiation on this point – no matter how much of a trusting relationship you have, no matter how much of a milquetoast you are in real life, even if she would swear on a stack of Bibles that she is 100 percent sure you would never hurt her in any way, there is no busting this kind of move without the two of you being in full agreement. This kind of sexual game can not, under any circumstances, be done spontaneously or incorporated on the fly during "typical" alpha male sex.

I'm going to start at the end on this one: After you've finished any sex involving a rape fantasy, make sure there is ample time to spend being very gentle, loving and tender toward your partner. It reinforces the fantasy element of what you've just done as well as the trust factor in your sexual relationship. It will also help you come out of what can be a very explosive and potentially addictive role for you.

When watching news stories about assault, portrayals in film of sex crimes, or even if a hot handyman comes over to fix the bathroom pipes, don't be a dick and make a joke referring to her fantasy. I'm sure you wouldn't dream of it, but I had to put it out there. It's very important that her fantasy stays in the comfort zone of your trusting, loving relationship and not connected to any real-life, dangerous scenarios.

I'd like to take this opportunity to bring up what we talked about before regarding the safe word – rape fantasies involve your partner saying no, fighting you off or even trying to escape from your grasp. It's part of the excitement, because these games start with her begging you to stop, and then begging you NOT to stop as she becomes aroused by being penetrated against her will.

So, understandably, you're not going to actually stop when she says, "Stop" or "No" or even "Ouch, quit it!" That's why a safe word that has nothing to do with your scenario needs to be agreed upon – as is the fact that you're to stop immediately and hold her gently, with no judgments.

What you DO want to do is elicit from her exactly what her fantasy entails beforehand, so that you can work together in building up to making it happen. Because force fantasies are pretty on the edge, you'll want to be experienced in a lot of non-forceful role-playing, depending on what she has in mind.

Again, depending on your woman and her fantasy, this can be quick or slow. Is it being forced to have sex for the first time by a high school love, or is it someone who barges into the house and throws her on the bed? Talk it out before anything is done at all, and let it have time to sink in.

After it's over and you've been tender with her – or whenever the time seems right – ask her what she liked and didn't like, and how you can improve on it. This will go a long way in reinforcing to her that you understand it was, in fact, just a game.

The most important thing to realize – for the both of you – is that it is perfectly normal for a woman to have a rape fantasy. (In a fantasy, the woman chooses the man, the scenario, the pace, etc. Plus, she has a safe word if she needs to end it at any time.) She is not bad or weird or damaged in any way simply because she has a fantasy about being raped. It's simply the alpha male desire taken to its logical, if most extreme, end.

IT'S NOT FUN UNLESS BOTH OF YOU ARE MUTUALLY SATISFIED

Given everything we have discussed, this is probably a good time to talk about the communication between you. I'd like to reiterate some points I have already made, but more importantly, I want to tell you how reading each other's cues can bring whole new levels of intensity to your alpha male lovemaking.

Verbal Communication

Here's a quick review of what we have talked about so far in terms of communicating with your partner when it comes to assertive sexual experimentation.

- It is normal for a woman to want her partner to be more forceful in the bedroom. There is nothing bad, wrong or even extreme about this type of desire or fantasy, nor does it mean that there is something wrong with the male partner.
- It is normal for most men to not be as forceful in the bedroom naturally, as

society has taught them to treat women with the utmost respect, and alpha male behavior might not lend itself to respectful behavior in their eyes.

- The woman needs to know exactly what her desires entail, and she needs to be able to express them in an open way. There are several ways she can go about this, from a sit-down conversation to after-sex pillow talk to being more forceful herself in bed to heat-of-the-moment requests.
- For any type of sex play involving a power dynamic, a safe word should be agreed upon. If it is spoken, the games should end and there should be a tender time followed by nonjudgmental conversation. (Then get back in the saddle and make some good memories!)
- Dirty talk is an important component of alpha male sex. Used by the man, it can supplement his actions and gauge her level of pleasure. Used by the woman, it can be a signal to him to go further, or to hold back.

Verbal communication does not have to be either a clinical discussion of the proceedings or raunchy talk that would make your mother blush. When the two of you are in the zone – meaning, when you're having a total connection with each other during your lovemaking – even a little comment made by one of you can send you both over the edge and into ecstasy.

When it comes to alpha male sex, this usually means an acknowledgement of the roles each of you are playing.

For example, let's say you're having some seriously rough sex. Guys, you're bending her six ways to Sunday. You have never seen her so turned on; you've never been more in love with her than at this moment.

Say it! With some extra hard thrusts, declare your love for her! "I've never been so in love with you than at this moment!" "I love being your man!" Whatever the spirit moves you to say is fair game – just keep it short.

And ladies, you can reinforce your appreciation for all that your man is doing by letting him know it! Tell him you'll never love another man. Tell him he's all the man you need. Tell him whatever you feel best expresses your love for him.

When this happens, often the vibe changes from one of "Hey, Honey, let's experiment" to two equals joined together, body and soul. What was a power game now is a passionate lovemaking that binds you together in deep, abiding love.

To be less sappy, there are other ways you can kick it up a notch, but while staying in the alpha male moment. A back-and-forth type of dare that acknowledges the game you're playing can allow you to connect on a relationship level as well as a sexual level.

"Can you take it?"

"Yeah, I can take it. Give me more."

"Oh, you want more, you're getting more. I'm going to give you something you'll remember all day tomorrow during that conference."

"I don't think you've got it in you."

"No?"

"No, come on, what are you waiting for, that conference is going to suck."

"Oh, I'll show you suck."

It balances the two worlds, and can lead to prolonged play between the sex and the talking, texting or other modes of alpha male play.

Non-Verbal Communication

However, not all of us are so verbose. In fact, many of us are not! While verbal communication is important in many facets of assertive sexual activity, it's not absolutely mandatory every single second. Sometimes, a simple glance, a wink or a nod can say what a thousand words never could.

It's all about reading each other. When you're in tune with one another, and you don't retreat off into your fantasy mindset, you can feel every weight shift, hesitation and rhythm change. You can hear each other's breathing, or the beginning of a gasp or a word that dies on the lips.

When there is that kind of connection, you don't need to talk at all!

Let's take a look at some examples.

- In Missionary position, and he is thrusting super hard into her. He's being very rough. All of a sudden, he gets nervous that maybe she's getting nervous about how rough it is. He slows down, holds back a little.

- She snaps to attention, locks into his eyes, and with a glance lets him know that she was loving it and he should keep going!
- She looks at him with a small "Thanks, this is better" look.

In a fraction of the time and with a minimum of embarrassment, they are on the same page again and all their worries are gone.

- How about the looks you give each other before you're ready for an orgasm? There is a bit of permission; a bit of the go-ahead; a bit of "I am about to give you a mind blowing orgasm" in these looks, the meanings of which are apparent in the subtle raise of the eyebrow or a squinting of the eyes.

- There is the warning look – the eyes bright, hard and locked in, NO. There is the "I love you so much" look. There are a million looks you can read on each other's faces, and you respond accordingly.

- Physical movements can give away so much, as well. The grasping hand going slack or holding on tight at the moment before an orgasm. The involuntary thrusting during orgasm, or the body-shaking shudder.

I'm sure you have experienced all of the above. If so, then this level of knowledge about your partner can only serve to intensify the alpha male sexual experience for both of you.

Whether it's seeing the mischievous smile on his face while he's ravishing her, or seeing a whole new level of ecstasy on her face because of what he is doing, being able to read each other is the best way to heighten the excitement when you're together.

BRINGING THE ALPHA MALE ELEMENT INTO YOUR RELATIONSHIP

I've gone on and on about how this kind of experimentation should not be allowed to bleed into your day-to-day relationship dynamic. But, there are a few things both of you can do to remind each other of your new, exciting sex life – while outside of the bedroom.

Guys, these are all up to you to initiate. Man up!

- If you're at a party, restaurant, bar or club and you find yourselves alone for a moment – say, in line for the bathroom, or in the foyer on your way out or in – grab her and give her a quick, passionate kiss. Then, let her go and resume a normal stance and appearance.
- Elevators! Quick-and-dirty make-outs in elevators are hot, hot, hot.
- Before she gets out of the car, grab her toward you for a passionate kiss.
- Did she just come out from getting ready, and she's looking hot? Tell her

in no uncertain terms, and tell her what it makes you want to do to her – also in no uncertain terms.

Ladies, you can let him know he's coming through with the goods, without launching into a lengthy discussion that is sure to take all the passion out of the game.

- Did he do something manly around the house? "Who da man?" followed by a saucy smack on the ass will make him feel like the king of the world.
- Make little comments about places you've had sex: "Well I don't want to put the vase there in case you decide to take me again on the table." Wink and smile, then move onto other things.

What Not To Do

Here are some ways that you really, really don't want to emphasize the alpha male sex you've been having.

Ladies: If he fails at doing something – say, if he can't make the DVD player work – don't say things like, "Well, I guess you're not an alpha male after all."

Guys: If you're not naturally playful with your lady, don't do things like slap her ass or grab her outside of the bedroom.

Guys: The same goes for what you might think passes for witty repartee. Don't joke about how you're the man of the house, and she'll do as you say. Those jokes are never, ever funny.

Ladies: Don't ever throw in his face that this was your idea. Emasculating him won't do him any good; it's not an incentive.

CONCLUSION

Congratulations! You are now on your way to becoming closer than ever by exploring this aspect of your sexual relationship.

I want to say again that a woman wanting her man to be more sexually assertive is not a reflection on an otherwise healthy relationship. It is merely a desire borne out of her ideas about femininity, power and sexual excitement.

Guys, if you are still confused, or hurt, or unsure about what this all means, I recommend you really take the time to listen to what your ladylove is telling you. Don't be afraid to ask questions, and get as clear as you can about exactly what she wants you to do, say or how she wants you to behave the next time you're getting busy between the sheets.

And ladies, don't be shy. Get what you want out of your sexual relationship. If he is not giving you what you need, then you have every right to let him know.

However, this is not the blame game; this is an attempt to make your sex life as a couple the very best it can be. That deserves respect, and mutual agreement as well as mutual satisfaction.

That last one – mutual satisfaction – is a big one. This is not just about what one partner wants, and the other one providing it. This does not have to be a sacrifice on anyone's part. Done right, the alpha male concept should be explosively titillating for both of you.

As a few words of parting advice, I'd like to encourage you to explore, discuss and, when possible, push the boundaries of your sexual relationship. There is absolutely no reason whatsoever to get into a rut sexually. There are literally a million and one things to do once that bedroom door closes at night, and I hope you discover every single one of them!

And do you know why? It's because sex is not just sex; it's another way of communicating with each other. It will strengthen your bond over all aspects of your relationship. It helps you to get to know each other even better, and to discover new things about this person you thought you knew everything about – the person with whom you are sharing your life, and your heart.

APPENDIX

TURN UP THE HEAT WITH SOME ROLE-PLAYING

Alright, we've gone over a lot of topics in this book, and I hope I've given you a full bag of ideas to try with your partner so the both of you can enjoy hot, spicy alpha male sex anytime of the day or night!

I'd like to go more into specifics about the ideas we've discussed, in case you're not exactly sure what's what when it comes to experimenting in the bedroom. And, if you're good, I'll throw in a couple of new ideas, too!

Earlier, I talked about the ability of role-playing as a way to overcome any awkwardness either of you might feel when experimenting with the power dynamic between the two of you. Now, let's take a closer look at what exactly goes into role-playing.

Basically, the two of you need to agree on a scenario that is exciting to you both. Other than that, it's all up to you how much you want to get into the details.

For some couples, it can be simply the talking that gets them into the mood of the role-playing game. Each person takes on their role, and "becomes" that person based on what they say. But for others, there can be costumes props, and even pre-arranged times at which they agree to meet as their characters.

Let's take the example of the handyman and the housewife. This is a popular one.

You could start out by simply making innuendos about him coming in to fix whatever is "broken" or to get out the "kinks" in your pipes. Or, you could go so far as to have her change into a housecoat and apron (with sexy lingerie underneath, of course!), and have him wear some kind of maintenance uniform (they are easily available for sale). Then, he can leave the house and come in as the handyman, with neither of you ever acknowledging your history or the fact that you've known each other a good long time.

You can knock on the door, and she answers and lets you in. While explaining the "problem," she can let her bathrobe slip open, or perhaps lean over in a suggestive way. There can be heavy flirting, but it should really be you initiating – being "rough trade," so to speak. Tell her what you think she "needs fixed," in no uncertain terms – and then, when the time is right, take her and have your way with her.

For professor and student, you might put on glasses and a suit, or she might carry some books. For boss and secretary, maybe she wears her glasses, and you're both in corporate attire. You might find a whole new use for that home office other than doing the taxes and paying the bills!

Teenager role-playing is also one that gets a lot of play. For many of us, those first sexual explorations are still the most exciting times in our dating histories – and a lot of those "tingly feelings" came from the guy wanting to do more or go further than the girl is comfortable with.

That's why I suggest the football star and cheerleader combination – it's simply the stereotypical high school characters. But you can make your characters fit whatever, and whomever, turned you on back in the day. You might even want to go to the local make-out point or lovers' lane with the car! Really get back into that time – the good parts, at least – and let yourselves be taken away with those feelings of first love. Play your favorite old make-out music, too, to get in the mood.

No matter what the scenario, it should play out like a porn film, basically: There is a ruse to the two of you being together in the same room, she is flirty, you get aggressive, and it ends with the tension and the passion levels so high that you finally have to take her and ravish her – and it can even be right there where you've set your scene.

The key to role-playing is never to break the mood. For the time that you're doing it, feel free to lose yourself in the moment and become that other character. Many, many couples have said that this helps them greatly in their sexual experiments.

And again, this is when you can hone your dirty-talk skills. By saying the things you want to say as your character, they can come easier to you and you can become more comfortable saying even the raunchiest things. Also, with role-playing, you can leave the dirty talk there in the scenario; it can be less embarrassing later, if you are someone who simply cannot get the hang of saying it with some spice.

A kind of role-playing can be done by renting a hotel room for the night or the weekend. People tend to feel unlike themselves in hotel rooms, as they are not surrounded by the things that remind them of their everyday lives. What better place, then, to lose yourselves in sexual experimentation?

Hotel rooms work great for client/escort fantasies, which can be a great way to break the alpha male ice. After all, if he is paying her to perform for him, he's going to get his money's worth by telling her exactly what to do, and how to do it!

Of course, it's not necessary to do this kind of role-playing when getting a hotel room. Sometimes it can just be a great excuse to get wild and rough and mess up the bed a bit. It really depends on what you are into.

The hotel room rendezvous works well if you agree to arrive separately. That way, she can be ready in bed for him, and he takes her the second he gets in the door.

Or, you can check in together, and start in the elevator on the way up. Then, once that door is opened, push her in the door and onto the bed and have at it. You can check out the room amenities later. Remember to put the "Do Not Disturb" sign on the door!

Another popular role-play scenario, especially for those just starting out with alpha male sex experimentation, is for the man to create a romantic, perhaps adventure-filled evening. Many women are surprised to find that romance plays a larger role in their assertive male fantasies than they had originally thought.

Or, while the evening may end up hot, rough and spicy as a jalapeno, it can easily start out with a great romantic evening – planned entirely by the man, with no input from the woman at all. This is a softer way, shall we say, for men to get used to "calling the shots."

It can also help the woman feel more feminine, and more amenable to receiving direction and other male assertive moves when it comes time to the sexual part of the evening's activities. This is especially good for the woman who has a high-powered job, or who is the head of the household – either financially, or in the day-to-day running of the house.

Guys, do it up right for a whole evening – and don't ask for a gold star for it, that's a big thing with women; they don't want it to be about you and this wonderful thing you did, they want the focus to be on them.

Hire a limo; rent a hotel room and order swanky room service; have a fire in the fireplace and Champagne on ice; have her follow a romantic scavenger hunt to the bedroom, where you'll be waiting. Just make sure you're directing it, every step of the way.

Feeling feminine and like the "weaker sex" is definitely a big part of the thrill for women in these scenarios, so ladies, do it up! Get out the sexy lingerie from the back of the dresser drawer. Shave, wax, exfoliate, perfume, spritz and spray until you feel like an irresistible goddess. It will go a long way in your fantasy of how the evening will go if you feel like you are absolutely, 100 percent ready to be seduced.

And speaking of seduced, this is another thing that is sometimes missing from the sexual focus of alpha male scenarios. Seduction has everything to do with sex, to be sure, but seduction can be used as a powerful male assertion when done correctly.

Bring some fun into your role-playing. It can be fun to meet in public, say, at a bar or restaurant for a date. Guys, show her your smooth moves with everything from ordering her drinks and maybe even her meal, to taking care of the check, or asking for a special dessert for her on the sly.

Ladies, let yourself be taken care of. Follow his lead, and see where the night takes you!

Another fun idea, particularly in this day and age of working couples, is for the woman to play up what I call the "June Cleaver" aspect of male authority. It's a good way to get the guy into the mentality of alpha maleness – by going back in time for an evening!

Dress nice for when he comes home from work. Have whatever his equivalent of "slippers, pipe and newspaper" is waiting for him when he comes in. Give him a backrub. Make his favorite meal. Ask him if there is anything at all you can do for him, and let him tell you – explicitly. Then he can "reward" you with big manly-man sex at the end of the night!

You know what's a sure-fire way to turn things up a notch, even though it's been talked about as such a cliché? Stripping games. I don't care whether it's poker, Yahtzee or Monopoly; the strip version of any game like this allows a playful element to come into the mix. Also, having him bring out his competitive streak, especially in such a manly game as poker, can really jumpstart his alpha male instincts.

Oh, and ladies? Make sure you lose, ok?

Lightning Source UK Ltd.
Milton Keynes UK
UKOW041941110113

204779UK00002B/236/P

9 781608 422982